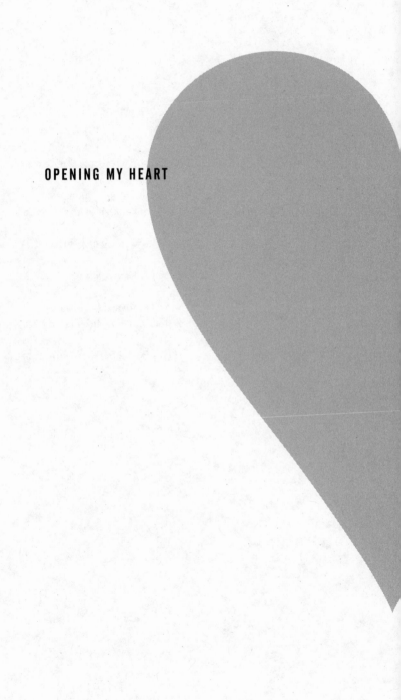

OPENING MY HEART

OPENING MY HEART

A JOURNEY FROM **NURSE** TO **PATIENT** AND BACK AGAIN

TILDA SHALOF

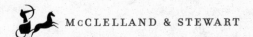 MᶜCLELLAND & STEWART

Library and Archives Canada Cataloguing in Publication

Shalof, Tilda
Opening my heart : a journey from nurse to patient and back again / Tilda Shalof.

ISBN 978-0-7710-7988-7

1. Shalof, Tilda—Health.
2. Heart—Surgery—Patients—Canada—Biography.
3. Nurses—Canada—Biography. I. Title.

RD598.S53 2011   362.197´4120092   C2010-906745-2

We acknowledge the financial support of the Government of Canada through the Book Publishing Industry Development Program and that of the Government of Ontario through the Ontario Media Development Corporation's Ontario Book Initiative. We further acknowledge the support of the Canada Council for the Arts and the Ontario Arts Council for our publishing program.

Published simultaneously in the United States of America by McClelland & Stewart Ltd., P.O. Box 1030, Plattsburgh, New York 12901

Library of Congress Control Number: 2010940066

Typeset in Filosofia by M&S, Toronto
Printed and bound in Canada

ANCIENT FOREST
FRIENDLY

This book was produced using ancient-forest friendly paper.

McClelland & Stewart Ltd.
75 Sherbourne Street
Toronto, Ontario
M5A 2P9
www.mcclelland.com

1 2 3 4 5   15 14 13 12 11

CONTENTS

Acknowledgements

Heartfelt thanks to the many people who took care of me and this book, especially:

Dr. Tirone David, Chief of Cardiac Surgery, Toronto General Hospital; Milutin Drobac, Pat McNama, Janet Morse, Len Sternberg, Ivor Teitelbaum, Joy Bartley, Maria Kirchhoff, Marion McRae, Leslie Moffat, Christine Sterpin; staff of CVICU and Cardiology 4A.

Judy Boychuk-Duchscher, Mary Ferguson-Paré, Doris Grinspun, Linda Haslam-Stroud, Paris Jalali, Mary-Lou King, Rosemary Kohr, Ruth Lee, Joan Lesmond, Marlene Medaglia, Judith Shamian, Laura-Lee Walter.

Marilyn Biderman, Elise Dintsman, Daneen DiTosto and family, John Fleming, Joy Friedman, Anna Gersman, Pamela Glass, Tex and Bonnie Shalof, Stephen Grant and Sandra Forbes, Robert Grant, Vanessa Herman-Landau and family, Omri Horwitz and family, Avery Kalpin, Annie Levitan, Solly Katz and family, Elba, Barry, and Nadine Lewis, Robyn, Bob, and Norah Sheppard and family, Michael and Barbara Turner-Vesselago, Chick and Dick Weiner.

The staff of the Medical-Surgical ICU at the Toronto General Hospital, the University Health Network, especially: Robert Bell, Lesley Barrans, Allyson Booth, Sherrill Collings, Nathalie Côté, Ingrid Daley, Belle Dhillon, James Downar, Gail Fairley, Maureen Falkenstein, Marcia Fletcher, Michael Fraser, Maude Foss, John Granton, Laura Hawryluck, Margaret Herridge, Grace Ho-Young,

Thileep Kandasamy, Brenda Kisic, Connie Kwan, Neil Lazar, Edna Lee, Vincent Lo, Murry Macdonald, Mindy Madonik, Bella Manos, Kate Matthews, Robert McGregor, Mercelies McHugh, Moira McNeill, Denise Morris, Wendy Radovanovic, Meera Rampersad Kissondath, Juliet Ramsay, Janice Stanley, Andrew Steel, Derek Strachan, Kelly Sundarsingh, Sharon Reynolds, Claire Thomas, Mugs Zweerman; The Critical Care Outreach Team; Arnie Aberman, Wilfred DeMajo, Brian Kavanagh, Stuart Reynolds.

Laura's Line: Lisa Huntington, Ann Flett, Cecilia Fulton, Judith Allan-Kyrinis, Mary Malone-Ryan, Linda McCaughey. The Bagel Club: Stephanie Bedford, Janet Hale, Jasna Tomé, and honourary member Amber Verdoni; Eric Bailis of St. Urbain Bagel.

All of Dr. Mehmet Oz's books have been helpful to me in improving my wellness and overall health. An excellent resource on cardiac surgery is www.heart-valve-surgery.com. *Shop Class as Soulcraft* by Matthew B. Crawford clarified my ideas about the value of hands-on work as it applies to nursing care. For the best writing teacher in the world, check out www.freefallwriting.com.

Everyone at McClelland & Stewart, especially Doug Pepper, Elizabeth Kribs, Terri Nimmo, Scott Richardson, Heather Sangster, Ashley Dunn.

Ivan, Harry, and Max Lewis – closest to my heart.

Note to the Reader

My heart was opened on an operating table and I knew that in order to tell this story, I would have to crack it wide open all over again. However, I am happy to do so if you will find something of your story in mine.

After twenty-five years as a nurse, I suddenly became a patient and was surprised to discover I had a lot to learn on the other side of the bedrails. Being in the hospital can be a confusing and frightening experience, even for me, a seasoned professional, entirely familiar with that world. What helped me the most was staying in charge of my patient experience and working in partnership with all of my caregivers. I show you how you can do that, too.

This is a true story. Details have been changed to protect privacy. Clinical information is accurate, but please consult experts about your medical issues. Don't pull some of the stunts I did: I didn't always make the wisest decisions about my own health care.

This book is for patients and caregivers (most of us will have the chance to be both at one time or another). I hope it is a comforting companion to anyone facing not just cardiac surgery but any hospitalization or illness. It's a lot to ask of a book, but many have done that — and more — for me.

Here's wishing you strength and courage to take care of yourself and others.

Tilda Shalof, RN, BSCN, CNCC (C)
Spring 2011

1

NO PROBLEM. I FEEL FINE!

The story of my heart begins with an earache in the night.

The ear belongs to my eleven-year-old son, Max, who wakes me, head in his hands, tears welling up. Sleepy mom and hard-boiled nurse that I am, I dope him up with a slurp of purple painkiller syrup and send him back to bed. But in the morning his ear still hurts and he's spiked a temperature, so I take him to the doctor.

The waiting room is packed. How much longer until our turn? I pester the receptionist, but she's too busy to answer. Hovering around the front desk, I scan the rack of doctors' business cards. Three general practitioners and an asthma specialist share this office. Oh, a cardiologist, too, and I pocket one of his cards. Some people collect stamps, antiques, or lovers. I collect cardiologists — a hobby of mine for years.

Eventually, we get to see Dr. Ivor Teitelbaum. He's my husband's doctor, and Max and his older brother, Harry's, doctor, but not mine. I don't go to doctors.

Ivor is a handsome, smartly dressed, young-looking middle-aged guy with an old-school manner. Always relaxed, he never rushes us along, despite the bustling waiting room. He examines Max, then offers me his otoscope so I can look into the ear canal myself and see the bulging, inflamed tympanic membrane, severe enough for Ivor to prescribe an antibiotic.

We get up to go, but I pause. "This cardiologist" — I wave the card at Ivor — "is he any good?"

"Very." He looks up from writing in Max's chart. "Who needs a cardiologist?"

I shoo Max back out to the waiting room, pull up my T-shirt, and nod at the stethoscope around Ivor's neck to remind him of my secret. I'd had to tell him so that my children's hearts could be checked for defects. Fortunately, neither inherited my heart problem.

It takes Ivor only a quick listen and then he looks up at me, hard, grips me by the shoulder, and steers me down the hall to the office of Dr. Milutin Drobac, the cardiologist.

"She needs to be seen," he tells the secretary, "as soon as possible."

"It's your lucky day," she says. "I just got a cancellation. Tomorrow at 11:00?"

"Sorry, I can't make it," I say. "I've booked a haircut."

She shoots me a glance. *What'll it be, your hair or your heart?*

Okay, heart it is.

At home I give Max the first dose of antibiotic and another dollop of grape-flavoured syrup. Soon he's back to his usual cheery self, so I hustle him off to school, leaving me alone to muse on my funny-sounding heart. *It's only a murmur,* I remind myself. What a cozy-sounding word. It almost sounds like a good thing to have. Who wouldn't want one? Many people have murmurs and most are normal or "innocent." *But not mine. Murmur* is a term that refers to any irregularity in the heart's blood flow, and in my case it's due to a serious heart defect – a faulty valve. It's congenital, meaning I was born with it.

As a child, I sensed something was wrong from the get-go. The heart specialists who spoke in solemn tones and the protective, cautious way my parents held me all conveyed the message: *Fragile – Handle with care!*

Then, around the age of ten, on one of many days off from school, I sat in a pediatrician's office and heard him say to my parents: "In time, her condition will worsen. One day she'll need open-heart surgery." He probably assumed I wasn't listening (a mistake many adults make around children) because my head was buried in a book. "No overexertion," he warned them, "and no sports or gym classes."

For my parents, that was a perfect prescription. It dovetailed with their need to keep me close, conveniently available to help my chronically ill and depressed mother. As far as they were concerned, school was optional.

Don't think I didn't hear the doctor's parting comment to my parents before he left the room: "A certain percentage of these children experience sudden death."

That's some experience, I thought and dove deeper into my book.

I've always known my heart could stop suddenly, but I banished the thought. I accorded my heart no respect, never allowing myself to think I had any physical limitations. I avoided strenuous physical activities, but in my mind, I was swimming the English Channel, riding horses, even running a marathon. Meanwhile, my parents became preoccupied with their own health problems and I became a nurse so that I could focus on other people's problems, not dare think of my own. My mo has always been to fly low on the medical radar and hope that an apple a day would keep the doctor away. (I eat a lot of apples.)

After a quiet, sedentary childhood, I threw caution to the wind and became a wild, adventurous teenager, then an active adult and energetic mother of two boys. I've always done whatever I wanted to do. That is, until recently. Lately, I haven't been feeling my best.

The next morning, I find myself where I always intended to never be – a cardiologist's office. First, there's the electrocardiogram (ECG) and an echocardiogram, tests I've helped many patients through, so I know the ropes. I strip off my T-shirt and bra, don the blue paper gown, jump up on the table, and lie down on my back. As Cezar, a big, burly guy who's Dr. Drobac's technologist, does the ECG, I glimpse the tracing over his shoulder, noting that my heart is in a regular rate of sixty beats per minute. *Normal sinus rhythm. So far so good.*

Cezar tears the printout off the machine and attaches it to my chart with a paper clip. For the echo, I flip to my left side so that he can obtain the best view. He glides the probe around my chest, digging it in at certain landmarks for a closer look, pausing, peering at the screen, then moving on. While Cezar works, I take a look around the small room, dimly lit as a nightclub to enhance the clarity of the picture onscreen. In the corner there's a treadmill for stress tests and a red "crash cart," equipped with defibrillator, pacemaker, and emergency drugs.

"Ever had to use that?" I point at it. *For a patient like me?*

"Yup." Cezar's brow creases, his eyes widen then narrow, but he keeps them trained on the screen in front of him. The sound of the amplified beats of my heart fills the room.

"See anything?" I inquire, well aware that he's not supposed to divulge anything, but I'm quite sure Cezar knows a thing or two. "Don't worry," I assure him. "You can tell me. I'm a nurse – an ICU nurse." He stays focused while I chatter on. "There's a problem with the valve, isn't there?"

Cezar pauses his probe and looks at me. "Big-time."

*But I feel fine! Well, maybe not my best . . ."*How bad is it?"

"I'll let Dr. Drobac speak with you about it."

I get dressed and graduate to the office of Dr. Drobac, who greets me warmly. As he reviews my ECG and echo report, I check him out. He's a tall, thin, elegant man who looks like he may have run a few marathons himself.

"You'll never see a fat cardiologist," my old nurse buddy Laura says. "Yet, there are many neurotic psychiatrists," she points out. Laura has developed extensive character profiles of every medical specialty. According to her, neurologists are precise and nerdy, gastroenterologists are messy and swear a lot — "think of what they do!" — and all ophthalmologists have small, legible handwriting. Her theories have yet to be tested.

Dr. Drobac introduces himself and we sit down opposite each other for the "functional inquiry," also known as the "patient interview."

"How have you been feeling?" he starts off.

"Great! No problem!" I say. "*Asymptomatic,*" I feel compelled to add.

"Any history of family illnesses?"

"My mother had early onset Parkinson's disease and manic depression. My father had type 2 diabetes and coronary artery disease." Died from it, too, but I keep that detail to myself so as not to prejudice my case.

"Do you smoke?"

"Never!" *How virtuous am I?*

"Take any prescription drugs on a regular basis?

"No." *My body is a temple!*

"How about recreational drugs?"

"No . . ." *Well, not lately . . .*

"What about alcohol?"

"Clearly, not enough." Now that gets a laugh out of him.

"Are you a Muslim?" he asks, breaking from the script of a standard cardiac history to figure out who I am. He hasn't quite got me pegged.

"No," I say. "Jewish. We like to eat. But I plan to start drinking more red wine as soon as possible. In moderation, of course. Strictly for the cardio-protective properties." *Broccoli and dark chocolate, too. From now on, I'm going to do everything right.* My mouth is dry, my hands are beginning to shake. "I have a feeling you're about to give me bad news."

"No, I'm not." He smiles. "Not at all."

Maybe it's nothing. What am I worried about? I feel perfectly fine.

"Any shortness of breath?" he continues.

"No . . . Not really." *Well . . . maybe, a little, now that you mention it.*

"Chest pain . . ."

"No, never!"

"What about chest discomfort or tightness, or racing heart-beats? Have you had any dizziness, light-headedness, coughing, or fainting spells?"

Now that you mention it. . . . I swallow the lump in my throat and stifle the harsh, dry cough I've had for a few months. Suddenly, I realize it is a *cardiac* cough. I'd have recognized it in a patient!

"How do you feel after you walk up a flight of stairs?"

"Not great," I admit. The truth is I haven't been able to walk up stairs for a few months now. I've been avoiding them when possible, and when not, I take them slowly, pushing against the heaviness in my chest, out of breath within moments. Ditto for hills and any inclines, for that matter.

"Do you have much stress at work?"

"Not at all." My patients do, but not me! But dare I mention that lately I can barely make it to the end of my shifts at the hospital? I am exhausted by lunchtime. "What's wrong with Tilda lately? She's always lying down," I heard a nurse say in the staff lounge the other day. "I'm taking a power nap," I said, popping up. At the end of my shifts, I've been dragging myself home and crashing into bed, not a drop of energy to spare.

"Are you able to do your daily activities at home?"

"Yes," I say but don't tell him that I couldn't rake leaves or shovel snow this past winter and the house is a mess. I move the vacuum cleaner two sweeps and have to sit down to rest. A laundry basket full of folded clothes sits at the bottom of the stairs, too heavy for me to lift and carry to the top.

"How about sexual activity?"

"Absolutely!"

"Sex is very beneficial for heart health," he explains.

In that case, I'll have sex every day—twice a day—if necessary! (Note to self: Notify Ivan of this new treatment protocol.)

"What about exercise?"

"I have a gym membership. I've done a few aerobics classes . . ."

Yes, I've showed up at all those classes with the improbable names like Guts and Butts, Cardio Funk, and Jazzercise. But my workouts have become lame and "half-hearted." I can't get my heart rate up above 100 and it takes a long time to recover and return to my resting rate. Oh, and I'll never bring a water bottle so I can have an excuse to keep stopping for a drink at the fountain to catch my breath.

"Are you keeping up with your peers?"

I haven't heard that phrase since I was fourteen when I begged my parents for the real Adidas running shoes with three stripes that the cool kids wore, not the cheap North Stars with only two. Of course it was only a fashion statement and status symbol, since I wasn't doing any running anyway.

Then there is my recent attempt to keep up — literally. It was on a vacation to Nelson, British Columbia, to visit my friend Robyn, during a group hike up a trail on Pulpit Rock, in the foothills of the Kootenay Range, near the Rockies — listed as a "gentle climb" in the guidebook. As I struggled to keep up with the pack, other friends easily strolling along faster, farther, and higher were casting back sympathetic gazes. Robyn stayed behind with me, looking worried.

"I'm taking it slow . . . so I can . . . enjoy . . . the view," I said as I huffed and puffed, shaky and breathless. *I need to make it to the top of this hill,* was all I could think as I kept stopping every few feet to clutch my chest, praying I wouldn't collapse on the way. *I'm a wounded buffalo, trying to keep up with the herd. Shoot the beast! Put it out of its misery!* We both knew something was wrong but didn't discuss it. Now I allow myself to know the truth: I could have dropped dead up there on that mountaintop.

Suddenly I realize the *real* reason that I quit the amateur parent-teacher talent show a few months ago. For my audition, I chose "A Cockeyed Optimist" from *South Pacific,* and mercifully they cut me off after a few bars since I sucked, but I was also too out of breath to finish. Nonetheless, they gave me a one-line solo in a song-and-dance number from *CATS* that required me to leap onto a platform wearing a skin-tight catsuit (what *was* I thinking?) and belt out, "Can you ride on your broomstick to places far distant?" I couldn't make it to *broomstick.* I bowed out, claiming to be too busy for rehearsals.

"So, no symptoms?" Dr. Drobac presses on.

"No." Only a premonition of doom, which I'm having right about now.

He makes notes in my chart — I now have a *chart!* — probably jotting down *unreliable historian,* the damning term for patients who aren't to be trusted. He's recorded my *symptoms* – what the patient reports – and now moves on to the physical examination, the *signs* – what he, the physician, observes and can measure.

We look at the ECG together. "Mild ventricular hypertrophy," he notes and points out the deep amplitude spikes in the chest leads and explains that my left ventricle is dangerously enlarged as a result of having to work extra hard to pump blood against the resistance of a constricted aortic valve. Any ICU nurse would grasp what he's talking about, but my thinking is so jumbled I can't follow his train of thought.

He stands up for the physical examination, ready to discover his own findings. Okay, let the objective tests be the judge. I may lie, but they won't.

Back in my patient "uniform," I lie down on the examining table. Dr. Drobac palpates my pulses, the carotid in my neck, brachial in my arm, radial at my wrist, femoral in my groin, popliteal at the back of my knees, and dorsalis in my feet. My pulses have always been weak and he notes that. He examines my jugular neck veins, which reflect the pressures in my heart. He places the bell of his stethoscope on my chest, closes his eyes, and listens. As I await my verdict I recall that according to Laura's profile, in addition to being slim and fit, cardiologists are the most musical of doctors. It does make sense: they spend their days listening to the melodies of the heart and have to be exquisitely attuned to pitch, volume, rhythm, tempo, crescendos, and diminuendos.

As Dr. Drobac moves his stethoscope around my chest, I know exactly what he hears: a slushy, mushy whooshing. My heart doesn't have the distinct sounds of a healthy cardiac cycle of contracting and relaxing; not the vigorous *lub-dub* of strong ventricles pumping effectively with valves opening and closing efficiently. My heart is the *swish, swish* of a lazy, burbling stream.

As a child, I was invited by medical schools as an interesting case study for doctors-in-training to learn abnormal heart sounds. Any first-year med student who could not correctly diagnose my obvious, loud systolic murmur would surely fail. But, when I grew up and became a nursing student myself, I stayed home from class the day they taught cardiac auscultation. We were supposed to listen to each other's hearts and my cover would have been blown.

Back in my civvies, I sit down with Dr. Drobac, who looks me squarely in the eyes. "It's clear why you've come to me now. You're not feeling well, not keeping up. The echo shows that your valve is tight. You have severe aortic stenosis." He gives me a moment to take that in, then says what I've waited all my life not to hear. "There is no doubt in my mind that you need open-heart surgery to replace your valve and to repair part of your aorta, too."

Valve plus aorta. Cut and blow-dry. Shave and a haircut, two bits.

The bottom drops out. I can't breathe. His words catapult me to the *other side.* I've crash-landed on Planet Patient, a destination where no one – but especially no nurse – wants to go. *Hey, don't I get any immunity from these things happening to me?*

Way over there is the doctor, talking to me from the safe side, waving and smiling from the far shore. He still seems to be thinking he's giving me good news.

"You'll need a cardiac angiogram first," he continues, eager to get this party started, "to rule out coronary artery disease before surgery. . . ."

Of course. The cardiac surgeon doesn't want to open me up and get in there only to find blocked arteries and that I need a coronary artery bypass as well as a valve replacement.

"Can this wait awhile?" I ask.

"Better to face it now, when you're feeling relatively well, with no other co-morbidities."

He means high blood pressure, peripheral vascular disease, coronary artery disease, hardening of the arteries, diabetes, kidney failure, a little of this, a touch of that, things waiting in the wings for most of us, one day, eventually.

"Your aorta is enlarged . . . the valve severely constricted . . . blood flow is reduced . . . ejection fraction is less than 30 per cent . . . you're not getting adequate blood supply."

"Could it be repaired? A minimally invasive procedure?" *Could this have been avoided if I'd dealt with it earlier?* That question, I wonder, but don't dare ask since I don't want to know the answer.

"No, your valve is too diseased. Extensive work needs to be done. It has to be replaced along with part of the aorta. It can only be fixed by opening the chest."

But these things happen to patients! "I need time to think about it."

"Don't take too long."

"When should it be done?"

"Soon. Within the next few weeks . . ."

Open-heart surgery — how inconvenient! I had lots of other, much more fun plans for the summer! Taking a break from my work in the ICU, spending time with Ivan and the kids, working as a camp nurse, spending time at my brother Tex's cottage on Georgian Bay. And this was the summer we were finally going to adopt a puppy, a year after the death of our elderly dog, Rambo.

Dr. Drobac asks if I have any questions. None and many, but first I have something to tell him that's way more urgent than any questions I might have.

"I want you to know that if I get a serious complication and don't wake up afterward, or if I become severely brain-damaged or have to be on prolonged life support, please let me go. If it's my time, let me go." *I do not want to be kept around beyond my useful shelf life.*

I blurt out these dire directives, not bothering to explain why catastrophe is uppermost on my mind.

He's incredulous, at a loss as to how to react to my at-the-ready disaster plan. "Have you thought this through?"

Have I ever! I think but can only nod yes to his question.

He looks perplexed, perhaps wondering how to reassure someone so anxious and somewhat irrational-sounding.

"If that's how you feel," he says, taking me at my word, "you should document your wishes and make sure to tell your family doctor."

"I don't have one."

"Get a lawyer and write a living will. Spell out your advance directives. Let your family know your wishes for your end-of-life care. Inform the surgeon." He shakes his head. "I don't want to disappoint you, but you're actually going to do very well. I wouldn't send you for surgery if I didn't think you were going to make it. This is a routine case."

Surely he's had patients who've died from "routine" surgery. And yes, I know, it is a good thing to be an ordinary patient with a common problem, but, see, I don't want to be a patient at all!

Walking slowly out of his office into the bright, hot summer afternoon, I'm scared out of my mind. Admittedly, there's a tiny bit of relief, too, to be set free from this heavy secret buried inside of me all of these years. In my heart of hearts, I knew this day would come. I've always felt I was getting away with something, continually dodging a bullet. Up until now, I've managed to stay on *this* side of the bed, a nurse in charge of others' care. Now I'll be the one *in* the bed, nurses bending over my body, tending to me.

I've always been such a big champion of our health care system, here in Canada, but will I remain a loyal fan when I'm on the receiving end?

I'm also a writer of stories that have been described as "heart-warming" and "heart-wrenching." The only thing I know for certain about the story ahead of me is that it will be heart-*stopping*.

2

EVERYTHING TO FEAR AND FEAR ITSELF

This is so not happening!

Oh yes it is.

I make my way out to the parking lot after seeing the cardiologist, my heart pounding, stomach churning, legs shaking. No "flight or fight" — I'm all *fright*. And I know, I know, I shouldn't drive, but I do, and worse, I call Ivan on my cellphone as I'm weaving in and out of traffic.

"We'll deal with it, Til," he says in his strong, confident way.

My news seems to come as no surprise to him. Ivan is an insurance broker and it always seemed odd that he never applied for a policy for me, but maybe he knew all along that I was too high risk to qualify for life insurance. Though we rarely talked about my heart condition, he must have realized it was serious.

At home, I drop my purse and keys and race to the phone. *I have to call Mary.* Mary Malone-Ryan. You can't get more Irish Catholic than that. But it's not her religion I need, it's her intellect — and her support. Originally from New Brunswick, Mary and I have been friends for years. We worked together in the ICU until she moved with her family to North Carolina, where she now works in a cardiovascular ICU.

"Til — eee!" Mary is ecstatic whenever I call, but in a split second she senses the worry in my voice and hers drops down. "Til-meister, what's wrong?"

She's shocked when I tell her. I'd kept this secret from everyone, especially nurse friends who would have insisted I see a doctor. Mary quickly changes gears, shifting straight into clinical mode, asking about my symptoms, blood pressure, electrocardiogram findings, and ejection fraction from my left ventricle. Once the data is out there between us, we both know there's no way around it: open-heart surgery is the only way to fix my problem.

"You can do this," she says calmly.

"No, I can't," I wail hysterically.

"You're strong, Tillie. Stronger than you think."

"No, weaker," I insist. I'm none of the noble things said about brave patients and their indomitable spirit, their courage. No one is going to call me a "fighter" or a "trooper"! I'm ready to run for the hills! I blubber on to Mary about putting my affairs in order, writing in-case-I-don't-make-it letters to my kids, and music for my funeral.

"Don't go there," Mary interrupts.

"Maybe I should delay the surgery. I feel perfectly fine."

"You're going to feel better afterward. You'll have so much more energy."

"If I make it."

"It's scary, but you're not going to die, Til."

"I'm just saying. It's possible. You know it is."

"Most valve replacements do very well."

Yes, most do, it's true, but some don't and those are the only ones I can think of. When I get off the phone with Mary, my mind turns to all the bad things that can happen. Patients who "don't do well" are the very ones I've dedicated my career to taking care of in the ICU. We're nurses. We know every possible Worst Case Scenario. WCSS are my specialty! Maybe I've gravitated toward caring for catastrophically ill people so that my problem would seem mild by comparison. Now my whole career seems like a preparation, a dress rehearsal – maybe even a death rehearsal? – for this. Waiting in the wings, I've played a supporting role, never the star. Now I'll be centre-stage. Or maybe it's more like I've been a loyal fan, a spectator at the game, always cheering the players from the bleachers. Now I'm going to be in the action, taking one for the team.

I can picture it all! The images come forth, unbidden, in full-blown technicolour, high-def, surround-sound: the whine of the pneumatic saw cutting into my chest, the crack of ribs, the whirr of the bypass machine, the bloody heart beating, slowing down, then still. When the heart is stopped there's a hush in the room while the surgeon works in silence.

Some things are better left unknown. It's scary enough even when it goes well. It's probably easier going through this as a civilian, but I don't have that luxury. We all fear the unknown, but it's what I know that scares me. I can't find comfort in "There's nothing to fear but fear itself" because there are real reasons to be afraid.

First, there are all the known, usual risks along with the unexpected, rare, or oddball events that end up as someone's presentation at a medical conference. Common complications are infection, ICU stress ulcers, deep vein thrombosis, which could lead to a pulmonary embolus (blood clot in the lung), burst blood vessels, uncontrolled bleeding, a blood clot or air bubble in the brain or in the heart itself, collapse of the lung (pneumothorax), or the dreaded acute respiratory distress syndrome, a devastating condition that causes massive lung inflammation, affects every organ, and carries a high mortality rate. There are iatrogenic problems (ones we cause) like unintended injuries or nosocomial (hospital-acquired) infections from inadequate hand-washing practices, contaminated surfaces, or even improperly sterilized instruments. We've all heard of such cases. Hospitals are dirty places. I know a patient who caught a Norwalk virus after a brief visit to the emergency department for a throat infection. (Why he went to the ER for a relatively minor problem is another story.) Hospitals are hotbeds of super-bugs such as methicillin-resistant staphylococcus aureus (MRSA) or Clostridium difficile (C difficile) floating all over the place. There are even infections specific to the ICU known by the Dr. Seuss-like mantra of "Zap the HAP, VAP, and DAP" – hospital-, ventilator-, and donor-acquired pneumonias.

More common than human error is the myriad ways your own body can let you down. Even if everyone does everything correctly, complications can happen. The immune system weakens and an opportunistic infection sets in. A bizarre reaction to an ordinary drug leads to the kidneys shutting down, boils all over the body, and the skin sloughing off. An unknown allergic reaction causes anaphylaxis, then cardiac arrest. I've seen all of these things happen. *For starters. That's on a good day.*

One day I was transferring a patient from the ICU to a step-down ward. She'd recovered from septic shock, pneumonia, and kidney failure. As I pushed the bed out of her room, I was chatting with her when suddenly she said, "My chest is exploding." On the monitor, I saw her heart rate go into an erratic rhythm and she quickly became unresponsive. Ventricular fibrillation! We did cardiac compressions in the doorway. We worked on her for more than an hour but couldn't save her. There were no indications this might happen and no one was at fault. Even an autopsy didn't reveal the cause of the cardiac arrest. Bodies break down. Not every problem can be prevented or fixed. Many times no one is to blame.

There are many unsolved puzzles like these, but there is also a logical cascade of events I've seen time and again. I call it "One Thing Leads to Another." A patient walks into the hospital with one problem and new problems are discovered – or caused. You start off with a straight-forward heart problem, then a respiratory infection sets in. An electrolyte disruption causes a heart arrhythmia. A "suspicious shadow" seen on the liver during a scan necessitates "further investigations," upon which another problem is revealed. A brief dip in blood pressure intra-operatively and next thing you know, the patient's gone into kidney failure and needs dialysis . . . and so on. What did I tell you? OTLTA.

I'll never forget a healthy, vibrant eighty-one-year-old grandmother who jogged five miles every day. At an annual checkup, her family doctor found hematuria, a trace of blood in her urine. A CT scan of her kidney showed a small mass. "It may cause a problem in ten years or so," a surgeon said, but the patient wanted to get it over with now when she was feeling well. A reasonable choice, yet, during the surgery, her intestine was accidentally nicked. In a few days, her peritoneal cavity was filled with fecal contents and her blood became contaminated. Meanwhile, the pathology report came back stating that the original kidney tumour was benign. She hadn't needed surgery in the first place, but now she needed multiple surgeries to drain the infection and to create an opening for feces to drain out. She got pneumonia, a hospital-acquired infection, then kidney failure.

A doctor's note in her chart read: *This patient is not a well woman. She was, once!*

She walked into the hospital in perfect health and by the time she left, she'd lost a kidney, most of her large and small intestine, had a chronic infection, and was bed ridden. After a year-long hospital stay, she was brought home and died there. Yes, I've seen too many times when it would have been best to leave well enough alone. Beware of OTLTA!

And we've all heard of the alarming incidence in hospitals of adverse events, sometimes called *medical errors*, which is actually a misleading term because it sounds like only doctors are capable of negligence or incompetence, but nurses can cause just as much harm – or healing, too. After all, nurses are the front-line care- givers, the ones actually doing most of the things that are being done to patients.

Every single day and night that we go to work, nurses live with the knowledge that our actions can hurt – even kill – a patient. Any nurse who forgets this reality should leave the profession. Immediately. Keeping the awareness of risk uppermost in my mind helps me practise safely. Most nurses have not made serious medication errors, but those who have will live with it all their lives. Yes, I have made a few medication errors. Thankfully, all were minor, didn't cause harm, and after full disclosure and an apology, I learned from them, but they haunt me still. However, I know some excel- lent professionals who couldn't come to terms with an error they'd made. They lost their confidence and ended up leaving the profes- sion, all because of one moment of inattention.

Paradoxically, my own "near-misses" have made me a better, more careful, and safer nurse. One trick I've learned is to con- stantly remind myself of all the things that *could* go wrong. For example, when I prepare and administer an infusion of heparin, a powerful blood thinner, I think how easily I could grab the black- topped bottle of 1,000 units per millilitre instead of the similar- sized, same-shaped, red-topped 10,000 units per millilitre. If I choose the black when it should be the red, the patient could receive too little heparin, possibly leading to a blood clot; if I draw from the red vial when the black is required, the patient will receive too much heparin, possibly causing bleeding.

Another mindset I use to stay safe is to read doctors' orders with a measure of caution and reserve, regarding each one as a *suggestion* or *recommendation* until I'm in complete agreement that what is ordered is the right course of action. Of course, in most cases it is, but if not, or if I have queries or concerns, I don't hesitate to speak up. When it comes to patient care, I'm not afraid to question authority or express my opinions, but it's taken me a long time to become like this. Am I going to feel as confident when I'm a patient as I do as a nurse?

Now right back at'cha! Payback time!

Yes, I know all the problems and potential for danger, but I calm myself down with the knowledge I have of all the hospital-wide efforts underway to fix them. Pre-mixed pharmacy medications, automated dispensing machines, computerized doctors' orders, a new culture of hand-hygiene awareness, and additional safety checks that are all in place are reassuring. However, nothing is foolproof, and none of these measures gives you an exemption from constantly thinking about safety.

For me, the best environment in which to be a patient or a nurse is one where there is a culture of safety and "no-blame." Not every nurse is as fortunate as I am to practise in such a "healthy" workplace, one that is as egalitarian and hierarchy-free as mine. It's a place where most people feel they can turn to a colleague and say, "Please double-check this dose for me" or "Hey, I think you forgot to ..." or "I'm not sure about this, what do you think?" No technology or inventions are going to prevent all mistakes because nothing can replace teamwork and old-fashioned vigilance. Safety is an

attitude, a way of doing things every bit as much as merely carrying out the correct actions.

The funny thing is, medical and medication errors are not
really uppermost on my list of fears. What scares me more is
another sort of "error" that is way more pervasive. There was a
time when I committed this kind of error myself. These are
instances when I saw a problem and did nothing. I looked away.
I'm only a nurse, I thought. *What can I do? They won't listen to me.
Someone might get mad at me. I might be wrong or get into trouble. I
might make a fool of myself.* Once, I overheard a nurse losing her
cool and speaking rudely to a patient and I kept quiet and didn't
intervene. Another time, a surgeon leaned over a patient's bedrails, his lab coat sleeve drooping into the patient's abdominal
wound. Afterward, he moved on to examine the next patient,
giving a free ride to those hitchhiking bacteria and stowaway
viruses and I didn't say anything. Not anymore!

Despite my fears – both the real ones and the irrational ones – I
know that my prognosis is good. My heart defect can be fixed. If all
goes well, I'll be "cured."

Ivan isn't fazed by any of this. In fact, in all the years I've known
him, I've seen him upset only a few times: at the murder of John
Lennon (yes, we've known each other that long), the horror of 9/11,
and moments in our marriage when I blurted out hurtful things. In
the evening after seeing the cardiologist, we sit together on the
couch and watch TV. Ivan reaches for my hand and gives it a squeeze.
At 11:00 he clicks over to the national news: terrorists, global
warming, and the economic crisis. At 11:30, it's over to the local
channel for a rundown of the latest stabbings, robberies, and
house fires around town. We drink coffee and go to bed. This is our
usual routine, crazy as it sounds.

Ivan lies down on the bed, settles in, and is soon sound asleep. I'm usually like that, too, but tonight I'm wide awake, listening to my heartbeats. *How many more will I have?* I get up and wander around the house, do a Sudoku puzzle, then go to my office and reorganize my bookshelves. Out in the kitchen, I open the refrigerator, hunting for a snack, but my usual emotional fix doesn't work. I can't eat a thing. I return to bed and see myself stretched out on a table, a magician's assistant ready to be cut in two. My heart springs out of my chest like a bird popping out of a Swiss cuckoo clock. They snatch it away before it can slide back in while scavengers scoop out my liver, kidneys, and brain, leaving me a hollow shell.

I spend the entire next day being anxious. It's all I have time for.

At night, I set the alarm to wake up so I can take my vital signs – make sure they're still vital. I drink water so I'll have to get up to pee, to know I'm still alive, like my father's corny riposte whenever he received an early morning phone call:

"No, you didn't wake me. I had to get up to answer the phone."

At 5:00, I'm wide awake, so I go to my office to stare at the books on the shelves. No longer the comforting and treasured friends I usually think of them, now they stand there and seem foreboding, as if they are taunting me with their solid longevity. They will out-live me. I may not get to read them all! Just yesterday I washed the cat's bowl and now it's the next day, already time to wash it again. Phoebe sits in the hallway, licking her paws, all of her purported "nine lives" intact.

I need to learn more about heart disease, specifically cardiac surgery, so I spend the afternoon consulting the experts – Dr. Google and Professor Wikipedia. They provide lots of information, some of it reliable, some not, and have terrible bedside manners. I consider myself somewhat of an expert on Bad Bedside Manner (BBM) because I have seen it all – and not just from doctors. The winner of the Worst BBM Award might be the radiologist who reviewed my patient's CT scan. A brain tumour was suspected, or possibly a cerebral bleed. "Is it serious?" the patient asked. "Yes," the doctor answered and then walked out of the room. The patient and I looked at each other in disbelief. A runner-up was the surgeon who came to speak to the parents of a twenty-year-old man. "Bad news," she said. "The pancreas is dead." (FYI: When speaking to families, the word *dead* should rarely, if ever, be used, especially when it is the *patient* who is dead.)

But in a way, bedside manner can be overrated. There's a specialist I know who is a superb diagnostician and an unerring clinician but is cold and impersonal with patients, arrogant and supercilious with everyone else. She has a chronic case of BBM. On many occasions after she's spoken with patients or their families, I have had to smooth things over or do damage control. On the other hand, if I ever get a disease related to her specialty, I will be running to beg her to be my doctor. Ideally, you'd get the whole package, but if I have to choose, I'll overlook BBM in a good doctor.

I tried to explain this to a friend who needs knee surgery and has been shopping for an orthopedic surgeon he can bond with. "I can't find the right one," he complains. "They're all carpenters. None of them takes the time to get to know me as a person. They just tinker with nuts and bolts." But a carpenter is exactly what you need! I tell him. A surgeon who is an expert craftsperson will fix your problem and make it work like new. If you want a friend, go somewhere else. Skill is what's needed, and when you get the personal touch on top of that, consider it a bonus.

No, there's not too much hand-holding going on in hospitals these days. Doctors may offer some in passing, but they tend to "come and go, talking of Michelangelo," a line from a T.S. Eliot poem that perfectly describes some doctors' detached, scientific stance. Whatever they offer in the way of comfort or encouragement is appreciated, but nurses are in a position to offer emotional support more intimately, consistently, and around the clock. (Whether they do so or not is another matter. We all know of cases when a nurse's anticipated Tender Loving Care turned out to be a Total Lack of Concern.) I guess I tend to cut doctors more slack about their BBM because they aren't usually at the bedside all that much. In the hospital, doctors typically spend a few minutes with each patient during the day (if at all) and rarely at night. It's nurses' bedside manner that is going to make it or break it for a patient.

By late afternoon, anxiety has overtaken me. My mind is spinning out of control, conjuring up more and more things to worry about. Frantically, I call Mary again.

"I'd be the same way," Mary says, "any nurse would."

By day and by night, I surf the net. Serendipitously, I discover that my obsessive behaviour is a diagnosis itself: cyberchrondria. I have decided to apply a few filters to my searches to avoid ramping up my terror more than necessary. I'll stick with reputable, evidence-based websites, and as for personal accounts, I won't read tales of fatal errors and screwups, botched jobs, horror stories of misdiagnosis and malpractice. I am able to interpret what I read, but what if I couldn't? A hockey mom on Max's team told me that after searching "heartburn" she diagnosed herself with acid reflux disease. When she went to her doctor, he said her upset stomach was a side-effect of an antibiotic she was on. A little knowledge can be a misleading, if not, in fact, a dangerous, thing.

Internet-surfing madness can take over if you don't use the information you glean judiciously. You have to make sure not to disproportionately emphasize some facts and overlook others.

You have to be able to glide appropriately from the general to the specific, from the theoretical to the concrete, and back again. Time and again, I have seen patients fall into these traps because they don't how to process certain information and understand how it relates to their specific situation.

But thankfully the days are long gone when doctors had the monopoly on information and were thought to own the knowledge and have all the "answers." Most doctors want to collaborate with patients, to forge a partnership, but too many patients confront doctors with bits of information, demands for tests or procedures, or raise objections to doctors' advice based on partial or inaccurate knowledge gleaned from the Internet. I'm going to try not to make this same mistake myself.

The first thing I learn in my Internet search is a loud wake-up call: heart disease, including coronary artery disease and other diseases related to the heart (such as valve problems), is the leading cause of death in North America. I am not alone.

Next, I review the heart's anatomy, its conduction system, and structures such as the arteries that supply its blood flow and the valves that control it. The aortic valve is one of four, in addition to the mitral, tricuspid, and pulmonic, and is positioned in between the left ventricle of the heart and the aorta, which sends oxygenated blood to the rest of the body, including the brain. Many people (1 per cent to 3 per cent in the sixty-five to seventy-five age group) develop calcified aortic valve stenosis (or narrowing) over time, but the most common congenital heart abnormality is exactly what I have — a bicuspid aortic valve. A normal aortic valve has three flaps, mine has only two. Over time, the irregularity becomes calcified, stiff, and constricted.

Then, echoes of the pediatrician's words: "Aortic stenosis carries a high risk of sudden cardiac death, especially when the ejection fraction is less than 35 per cent." *Mine is 30 per cent!* A normal ejection fraction is 50 per cent to 70 per cent; it represents the portion of blood volume ejected from the heart with each heartbeat.

As for second opinions, in my particular case, there is a consensus. If left untreated, my heart condition will only worsen. "Once a patient becomes symptomatic, the likelihood of sudden death within a year is more than 50 per cent." Furthermore, cardiac arrest in the patient with aortic stenosis resists all resuscitation attempts. (Well, sudden death has got to be preferable to the slow, tortuous deaths I've witnessed in the ICU. Here's my chance to find out.) There is no medical treatment for my condition, only surgery will correct it. Want to know the most common risk factor in heart disease? It's denial. (Sound like anyone you know? I guess I'm not in denial anymore.) "Without surgery, three-quarters of patients die within three years of symptom onset."

But there's good news, too: "Surgery restores a normal life expectancy and improved quality of life in the majority of patients." And there's a great deal of comfort to be found in the patient blogs that offer information, companionship, and commiseration. Reading other people's posts, I feel part of a supportive community, even though their stories range from reassuring to disturbing. There are inspiring accounts of patients who've gone on to run marathons and climb Mount Everest alongside reports of debilitating cardiac depression and post-traumatic stress syndrome in which they experienced disturbing flashbacks and nightmares post-operatively. Sprinkled throughout are interesting tidbits such as the blogger who received a pig heart valve from a surgeon named Dr. Swineheart (!), a chatroom group discussing the challenges of finding a comfortable bra after cardiac surgery (front-closing is best), and a posting on eBay (with several

bids) for a prosthetic heart valve – now that's extreme DIY! I discover that California governor Arnold Schwarzenegger had a
valve replacement – ditto for hockey player Teppo Numminem,
a defenceman for the Buffalo Sabres who now, a year after his surgery, is back on the ice, re-signed with the team.* Another interesting factoid: my clever strategy of stopping to chat or feign
interest so that I can catch my breath is a compensatory mechan-
ism called *schaufenster shauen,* apparently used by many ingenious
cardiac patients!

Everything I read corroborates what Dr. Drobac told me, but I
know sometimes doctors withhold information so as not to worry
patients. "Don't ask, don't tell" can be their MO. They may give a
soft spin, keeping back certain details. But the Internet doesn't
hold back. It lays it out there in a harrowing onslaught of TMI –
Too Much Information. It makes me waver between thinking,
"Ignorance is bliss" and "Knowledge is power." I've gone from
wanting to know nothing to devouring as much information as
possible. The more I read, the worse I feel, yet I forge on, trying to
stay on reliable, evidence-based sites.

Other than Mary, I don't feel ready to tell anyone else – especially
not Vanessa, who is also a very close friend but coincidentally is
dealing with her husband's heart problems right now. Steven's
heart was damaged by radiation he received years ago for cancer. I
don't want to add to her worry, yet I knowingly added to his when
I visited him in the hospital a few months ago.

"I have something wrong with my heart, too," I blurted out, suddenly compelled to share my secret with him, feeling certain he
would understand.

---

* Other celebrity heart valve patients include actor Robin Williams, former First Lady
of the United States Barbara Bush, and journalist Barbara Walters. I'm in good company.

"Take care of it," he said. "You have something that can be fixed."

Not like me, he didn't say. That was two weeks before Max's ear infection, which has long since resolved. Needless to say, my problem hasn't, nor has Steven's.

As for other friends, I can't tell them. Robyn will worry and Joy will be critical and unsympathetic. For years, she's been nagging me to take better care of myself. She goes for annual checkups, watches her weight, exercises, and is always popping vitamins and supplements to improve her "wellness." Nine years ago, when we both turned forty, she had a bone scan, a colonoscopy, and a mammogram. The results were normal, but she still keeps shopping around for new doctors who will do more tests and is constantly jonesing for more medical procedures and blood panels.

"You're abusing the system. Our health care system is in dire straits because of you," I tease her, but she points out that it's only responsible preventive health care and I can't argue with that.

By the afternoon, I am positively *google*-eyed so I take a break. In a fleeting interlude of sanity, I review my "past medical history" (the inane redundancy reminding me of my father's oft-repeated comment: "Where else would history be but in the past?") Believing that most things get better on their own, I rarely go to doctors. Most nurses are like this. We're level-headed, pragmatic, generally optimistic types who don't tend to think the worst. We're more likely to take things down a notch, not jump to the conclusion that a cough is pneumonia or a headache a brain tumour. We brush these things off, saving ourselves for the real, big-time problems. Maybe it's because we've been exposed to medical problems that are so much worse that we are grateful for everyday aches and pains. In fact, most of us have a rather skewed perspective because of our work. There are times when I've been in a group of people at a concert or on the subway and look around in amazement, marvel-

ling that none of them are intubated, unconscious, or hemorrhag-
ing. *Wow, most people are healthy,* I am reminded.

Myself, I'm the opposite of a hypochondriac; I think every little
pain or discomfort is nothing rather than *something*. I stay away
from doctors. Don't get me wrong, I have worked with hundreds of
them, many of them excellent, a few outstanding. I respect them
and trust them, but for myself, I keep clear of them or choose ones
who tell me what I want to hear, like an elderly cardiologist I went
to see many years ago. He prophesied that by the time I'd need
cardiac surgery, they'd be doing it with laser beams and robots. He
has since retired, but I've ridden on the prediction of that *Star
Wars* era at which we are now at the forefront. Yes, many heart
problems are being fixed that way, without using big knives, but
not mine, not yet.

Now it's finally time to come clean with my own health history
and face up to the fact that I'm not exactly a "virgin" patient as I like
to think of myself. Here we go:

A few years ago, while I was working in the ICU, I was sprayed in
the eye with lung secretions from a patient who had HIV and was
hepatitis C positive. I was freaking out and in my terror kicked up
quite a ruckus in my hospital's ER. "I must be seen immediately," I
demanded. "I've been exposed to biohazardous material!" When
that didn't work, I reminded them that I worked here and had
patients to take care of.

Yeah, let me get back to risking my life in this dangerous job!

They wouldn't budge. I would be triaged just like everyone else,
and since I wasn't bleeding, unconscious, or having chest pain and
the place was hopping busy, it would take a few hours to be seen. In
case you don't believe that I didn't get special treatment, while I
was waiting to be seen I happened to catch sight of the brilliant
physician with the BBM, walking down a corridor outside the ER.

Maybe she can move things along! I called out to her. She looked back, but at first glance all she saw was a patient in a hospital gown. When she recognized me but realized that my problem involved my eye, not the part of the body she specialized in, she lost interest and waved goodbye.

No longer enjoying any insider status, fuming, I settled down to wait along with the rest of the walking wounded. In due course, I was seen by a doctor, my eye was irrigated, and I was given a tetanus booster and my hepatitis titers were tested. For the next year, I had monthly baseline blood work, was checked for signs of infection, and did lots of worrying but fortunately didn't get sick.

Years later, I was a more reluctant patient when I became pregnant. At a pre-natal checkup, a doctor listened to my heart and sent me straightaway to a high-risk pregnancy clinic. When I protested what I saw as his excessive caution, he gave me a stern reality check. "You could get into serious trouble, go into heart failure or cardiac arrest. Your baby might not receive enough blood supply or oxygen."

Oh. I hadn't thought of that. Never mind.

Luckily, all went smoothly during the birth, and both times my babies were healthy. However, as I was leaving the hospital, two days after the birth of my second baby, the obstetrician warned, "You need to be followed by a cardiologist. Your valve is getting worse."

A day later, at home, I felt terrible – I had never felt so unwell. True, I was exhausted, but isn't every new mother? Harder to explain away were my swollen ankles and the difficulty I had sitting and breathing. When I listened to my chest with my stethoscope and heard the wet crackles in both of my lungs, I knew I was in congestive heart failure. Fluid from my heart was backing into my lungs. I swallowed a few Lasix tablets I had stashed away, which I kept on hand in case of just such an occurrence, and took it easy, laying low for a few days until the diuretic got rid of the excess fluid my heart couldn't handle.

[Public Service Announcement: Do not try this one at home, folks. Don't do as I did. Seek treatment from a doctor or other health care professional if you are in congestive heart failure. It's a medical emergency.]

That was twelve years ago and I can't believe I've made it this far with a heart like mine.

Then there was an evening, two years ago, working in the ICU with Cara, a young, pretty nurse fairly new to the ICU at the time. She was busy with her patient on the one side of the room, and I was busy with mine on the other, when two things happened. My patient, a seventy-two-year-old man, three days post-op thoracic aneurysm repair, became violent and confused. At the very same time, a sharp pain rose up from deep inside of me and grabbed me at my back.

"Those guys next door . . . Tell them to deal me in! Now!" my patient shouted at me from his bed. I clutched my side as he craned his neck, trying to peer into the next patient's room. The pain was sharp. *Yikes, what is this?*

My patient pulled at his IV tubing, then yanked it out of his vein. "I'm out of here," he yelled, throwing off the covers and banging on the siderails. Dark red blood splattered his sheets. "Give me my balloon! I'm going to the party." He grabbed so hard at the IV tubing that the pole toppled to the floor with a crash. Luckily he had sedation ordered and had another IV site in his neck. With shaky hands, I drew up five milligrams of Valium in a syringe and made my way over to give it to him. *If I can get him calmed down, I can figure out what's wrong with me.*

He eyed me warily. "If you come near me with that, I'll scratch your eyes out." He fumbled around with his arterial line, then in one fell swoop ripped that out, too. Now, bright red blood was pumping out from his artery, spraying in an arc around the room.

I retreated to my side of the room, panting with pain that was by then excruciating. *He'll bleed to death without pressure on that artery.* I called over to Cara for help, but she had already come running when she heard the IV pole crash. "Take over for me!" I yelled. I had no choice but to leave her alone with two unstable patients, one of whom was combative. As I staggered down to the emergency department, lurching along hospital corridors and vomiting into a plastic bag, I heard, "Code White, Code White, Medical-Surgical ICU" over the loudspeaker. It means a violent patient and summons the security guards to help out. I prayed that guy hadn't attacked Cara.

In minutes, I'd gone from a walking, talking nurse to a flat-out, full-blown patient. I even looked the part in my ICU scrub pants and a hospital-issue gown.

An ultrasound showed a kidney stone. A nurse started an IV and injected one milligram of morphine for the pain and an anti-emetic for the nausea. Ahh, relief came in moments. After a few hours, I passed the stone. I felt great, good to go.

I put the incident out of my mind until about a year later. I awoke during the night with a start, certain I was being stabbed. It was the same searing pain but now on the other side. *It'll pass, just like the last time. Ride it out. Don't go to the hospital!*

Within an hour, the pain escalated. I was frantic. "Take me to the hospital," I begged Ivan and he drove me to the nearest one. In the car, I writhed and moaned, tried to stand up on the seat, even considered jumping out. I have known patients who bore their pain with great dignity, but I had none. I was the opposite of dignity. Pain turned me into an animal.

At the hospital, there was the usual chaos and desperation so familiar to me that it actually calmed me down. All the seats were

taken, people were standing around sipping coffee, leaning against
the walls. It was any Toronto scene with hijabs and backpacks, tur-
bans and jeans, jallabeyahs, saris, and dashikis. It was also any ER
scene: a gaunt, bald woman draped with a homemade, brightly
coloured crocheted afghan, sitting in a wheelchair vomiting into a
basin; a biker dude in black leather and studs bleeding from slash
wounds on his arms and neck; a red-faced baby crying in its mother's arms. Even the requisite drunk who was in a room by himself,
screaming, "I'll kill you, Mommy. You'll be dead in three days!"
Ho-hum. Another day at the office. To me, the only thing that mattered was my pain.

It looked like it was going to be a long wait, so I sent Ivan home
to look after the kids while a triage nurse listened to my story, took
my vital signs, and sent me back out to the waiting room. I knew
the score: in my street clothes, I was a civilian like everyone else. I
found a plastic chair jammed up beside a vending machine, sat
down, and waited. The pain came in waves. I moaned and groaned
with the rest of them.

A nurse appeared and one man called out, "I'm dying, I'm dying!"

"Wait until the doctor sees you," she said. "He'll decide if you're
dying or not."

"Let's try another hospital. It's taking too long," said a young girl
pulling on her boyfriend's arm. How serious could her problem
be? (Or was he the one with the problem?) I'd seen them smooch-
ing hot and heavy in the corner just moments ago.

After those two left, the group of us that remained kept up one
another's spirits. We began to bond. When someone was called in,
we cheered and gave them high-fives. I joked that after this, we
should all be friends on Facebook.

"What are you in for?" I struck up a conversation with a fellow
inmate—I mean, *patient*—a guy in his twenties who'd cut his finger

slicing potatoes and had a superficial wound. That happened last night and now his entire hand was red and swollen.

"Thought I'd come in, get it checked out," he said cheerfully.

"May I?" He nodded and I felt his hand, wrist, and arm — all warm. I took a pen out of my purse. As he spoke on his cellphone to his girlfriend, I drew a border outlining the inflamed area that reached to his wrist.

We sat. One hour, then two. Patients came and went. Paramedics rushed in with a motor vehicle accident victim. I went over to watch the action on the sidelines. When I returned to my seat, I took a look at the guy's hand. The redness was extending beyond the line I'd drawn at his wrist, to his arm.

The triage nurse came out. "Telda Shalcot?" she called out.

Close enough. I got up to go in, then stopped short. I was in pain, but this young guy had a rapidly advancing skin infection that could be potentially life-threatening. In a few hours the bacteria could be in his bloodstream and he'd end up in the ICU, unconscious, septic, and on life support. Why didn't this nurse see what I saw? Too busy to see the obvious?

"Take him next," I told her. The other patients looked at me in awe. *A saint in their midst!*

"Suit yourself," the nurse said. I returned to pacing and tried to distract myself by reading the posters plastered on the walls. "Your Pain Matters to Us" and "Pain Is a Corporate Priority." No one around here seemed to be feeling my pain. One poster explained triage: "Along with major injury, no pulse or breath, unconsciousness, bleeding, shortness of breath at rest, unmanaged, severe pain is a medical emergency." My pain was an emergency to me. *The others have a low-pain tolerance. They're exaggerating. They say it's bad, but trust me, mine is worse.* I once knew a nurse who was a midwife (he was male so "midhusband"?) from the Philippines.

He told me he used to offer women in labour two Tylenol and they were grateful for that. "I hope it was extra-strength," I kidded him.

At last, salvation came and her name tag read "Emma, R.N." in cartoon letters, with her surname crossed out. (I've never understood the reasoning for this. Nurses say it's to prevent stalkers, but how likely is that? Do we really need protection from each other and does hiding your name give it to you? I guess these days, everyone feels vulnerable in the hospital, nurses as well as patients.) Bent over in pain, I trailed in after Emma, who walked briskly ahead of me. She directed me to a cubicle with a stretcher and handed me a hospital gown. She looked bored, like, *Get me out of here.* I know how to take care of myself in hospitals, so I didn't need her bedside manner, but what about real patients who did? In the hospital, emotions can become so heightened that a nurse's mild indifference feels like cruelty. Likewise, for frightened or anxious people, common courtesy can come across as extraordinary compassion. "Thank you for your extreme kindness," a family member once said when I accompanied them into the ICU for the first time; they felt my ordinary gesture so keenly.

"How's your pain?" Emma asked as she was about to leave.

Here's what I know about pain in hospitals: whatever dose or frequency of whatever drug is ordered, it all comes down to a nurse's mercy; it's in a nurse's hand. In school we learned that *pain is whatever the patient says it is; pain is the Fifth Vital Sign* (after pulse, blood pressure, temperature, and respiratory rate); *doctors under-prescribe and nurses under-administer.*

On a scale of one to ten, my pain was a nine a few minutes ago, but now it's a seven. Another spasm will probably hit me in a few minutes so should I play it safe and say nine, or should I conserve my points and say six? Better to keep eight or nine for later, but what if Nurse Emma's not around then?

"Seven – seven and a half," I equivocate. "The Russian judge gives it an eight."

She didn't find my joke funny, so I figured I'd better stop kidding around or she wouldn't take my pain seriously, even though humour was the only way I could endure it.

"I'll get you something," she said and then disappeared behind the curtain. An hour passed. The pain came and went, but Nurse Emma didn't. I got up to find her, and another nurse told me she'd gone on a break. "I'm having pain!" I announced loudly at the nursing station, then retreated to my cubicle. Eventually, Nurse Emma showed up.

Her total indifference was maddening. I was embarrassed we were even in the same profession, but I decided to put her on notice. "I'm a nurse, too." *My eyes are on you.*

"Cool." She prodded my arm. "Your veins are bad."

"Sorry about that." I pointed out a possible candidate, from which she drew blood quite capably. She started an IV and hung a small bag of saline running at a slow rate. "The doctor will see you soon." As soon as she left, I reached over and sped up my IV. *I need more fluid to flush out the stone. This nurse doesn't know her ass from her elbow!*

A few minutes later, the doctor came in and the first thing he said was, "Whoa, this patient is getting too much fluid!"

"I had set it at a slower rate." Nurse Emma glared at me as she adjusted the IV.

"It's true, normally, you'd push fluids," the doctor explained to me, "but not when you're in the midst of passing a stone. One kidney might be obstructed and become swollen while the other continues to produce urine."

Oh, snap! Hydronephrosis. Who's the bad nurse now? I would hate to have me for a patient. Then, just as he was about to order a dose of that magical morphine, he paused. "Any past medical history?"

No, I said, in no mood to quibble about the inane redundancy, only pray he wouldn't examine me, which might involve listening to my heart with his stethoscope. Luckily, he didn't bother. Soon, the narcotic kicked in and I dozed off. When I woke up, I went to the bathroom and heard a tiny, metallic-sounding clink in the toilet bowl. With a vinyl glove I'd nabbed from the clean utility room, I fished out my prize and held it up for examination. How proud I felt at what I'd produced. Famished, I was ready to reward myself with a nice lunch. I returned to my room and waited for them to discharge me.

I waited. No one came. My IV ran dry and clotted off. I took it out myself, then tidied my room, stripped the bed, and remade it with clean sheets I helped myself to from the linen cart. After dumping my hospital gown and linen into the laundry basket, I was ready to leave. As I walked past the nursing station I overheard a doctor. "We cured her. It's a miracle." I chuckled at his little joke. It was exactly the kind of thing I would have said had I been on that side of things.

Now, in the interests of full disclosure, I should mention that, yes, I told Dr. Drobac that I don't have a family doctor, but I lied about that, too. I do have one – a very good one, in fact. Dr. Janet Morse is smart, wise, kind, and always makes time to see me. A few years ago I went to her for something minor and she pointed out that I was long overdue for a checkup. I heartily agreed. She booked an appointment and I called the next day to cancel it. Coming to her now, she may not be so agreeable to take on a "non-compliant" patient like me and I can't say I blame her. But she welcomes me back warmly. When I tell her about my visit to the cardiologist she looks concerned. I wonder if she feels a twinge of liability for not insisting I be followed sooner. I rush to reassure her. "I neglected my health. You bear no responsibility whatsoever."

She reads me every bit as accurately. "Nor do you. You didn't cause this. You did nothing wrong. This defect was something you were born with."

But I worry that I may have made it worse by leaving it so long. She senses that I'm feeling at fault, and faulty, too. It's my own hangup because last night when I apologized to Ivan for this disruption to our lives his look of surprise told me he didn't see it that way. Ivan doesn't waste time wishing things were other than exactly the way they are. As for our kids, I'm not ready to tell them, not yet. Of what use is a sick mother? That's what I had and I vowed never to be that to my own kids. Over the years, I've done everything possible to stay healthy – except for taking care of myself, that is.

Dr. Morse orders blood work, and this time I promise to go.

Later, at home, back on the phone with Mary, I let it rip. "What if my heart doesn't start up again?" *The key is in the ignition, but the motor won't turn over!*

"That never happens," Mary scoffs, "but if it does, they'll put in a pacemaker. Tillie, you're going to make it. It's not your time to go. God has a plan for you."

Many people automatically utter such pious phrases, but Mary actually means them. She is sincerely religious, a devout Catholic who doesn't mess with the Third Commandment – or any of them, for that matter.

"At least you don't have to worry about medical coverage," she says on a more practical note. Living in the United States, it's new for Mary to have to think about health insurance. Yes, it's true. There are lots of things to worry about when you're facing open-heart surgery, but how I was going to pay for it wasn't one of them.

The next morning, Mary calls back.

"Tillie, I just got home from night shift. My patient was a seventy-two-year-old woman, twenty-four hours post–aortic valve replacement. As soon as we extubated her she was raring to go, practically jumping out of bed. She told me, 'You call your friend, dearie, and tell her not to worry. She'll be okay.'"

Up until now, nothing has cheered me, except this, a little.

3

FEARLESS NURSES

Night shift.

I have to be a nurse again, one last time before going off to camp, and then who knows when I'll be back at work?

"Should you be doing this?" Ivan asks as he watches me getting ready. He seems worried about me – or maybe about the patients who will be in my care – but, as I tell him, I need to do this. I leave the house around 6:30 in the evening – or 1830 hours – and drive downtown for my shift, which starts at precisely 1915 hours. On the way, I turn on the *Saturday Evening Golden Oldies* and listen to the Four Seasons sing "Big Girls Don't Cry" and Elvis croon "It's Now or Never."

Welcome to Toronto General Hospital, my world. Affectionately called "The Big House" by insiders, this huge, venerable medical centre is a mecca of world-class research, academic teaching, and exemplary patient care (according to the corporate mission statement) that specializes in cardiac surgery, organ transplantation, the treatment of eating disorders, and stem cell research (among other things). It has also been my place of work for eons and I have always felt proud to work here. But now, entering the revolving front door and standing for a moment in the main lobby, I see it with new eyes and am reminded that most people don't like hospitals. (I guess I forgot.) Not too much *hospital-ity* around here or many friendly faces or smiles, especially this late in the day when everyone who doesn't have to be here is scurrying off in the opposite direction, heading home. People coming in are reluctant and frightened; those leaving are eager and relieved. *No one wants to be here!*

In the hospital, everything and anything can happen – and frequently does. Nothing that goes on here surprises me. I've seen it all – birth, life, and death – in all its variations – not to mention sex, drugs, and rock 'n' roll. Every human emotion and activity takes place here: fainting, yelling, joking, sobbing, laughing, doctors crying, nurses dancing; gentle folk raise their fists, the cheerful become melancholy, and the timid learn to be outspoken. A patient gets married moments before dying. A son donates a lobe of his liver that saves his mother's life. A woman swallows the contents of her medicine bottles and we race to rescue the life she's tried to escape. A man breathes easy for the first time, now with new healthy lungs, a gift from an unknown family. No, it's not an episode from a television show, it's any day – or night – in a big-city hospital.

If you walk these halls and take a peek into the rooms you will see grim, ghastly sights. You'll smell the pungent mix of bodily fluids and industrial-strength chemicals. You'll hear people calling out in distress or confusion, and sometimes their cries go unanswered. Like a prison or a battlefield, the hospital is every bit as raw and extreme. You will be reminded that human suffering is close at hand; you don't have to travel to faraway places to find it.

I feel right at home here. It's my comfort zone. Hospitals are my second home; they're in my blood. As a child, I accompanied my parents to their numerous doctors' appointments. As a teenager, I spent my summers as a volunteer "candy striper." Years later, I resurfaced as a student nurse, and for the past twenty-eight years, I've been showing up, taking care of patients, and still trying to figure out the mysteries of this world, as a nurse.

I have stayed the course, working during the profligate 1980s, laid off suddenly in the mean, restructuring 1990s, when there was no "job security" and the joke was, "Don't bring a lunch." Eventually, I was rehired to do the same job and have remained employed here throughout these sober, downsizing times. Because I've been in it so long, I'm often asked the question: What has changed?

A lot.

Back when I was a teenager spending summer vacations in hospitals, strolling the wards, pushing a blue cart filled with books and magazines that I handed out to patients, I would stop to sit on the edge of their beds to chat and joke around. It's a different reality now. There's a huge shift. These days, hospital patients are not reading novels. They're too sick. Patients who are deemed "stable" or sometimes merely partially recovered are sent home to be cared for there – or not. The ones who remain in hospital have complicated, chronic medical issues, are unstable, often older, and need a great deal of complex nursing care. They have multiple IVs, are on oxygen, many have wounds and are receiving invasive treatments. (I have heard of hospitals in the United States that offer gourmet meals and spa treatments in order to improve "patient satisfaction." Want my advice? If you are well enough to enjoy such things, stay home.)

People are in the hospital because they need nursing care, and too often there aren't enough nurses to do the job properly. We all know of cases of patients who needed more nursing care than they received. "I rang the call bell and no one came." "I didn't see a nurse all day or night." Then there are worse tales of insufficient monitoring or inattention to serious problems.

All true, but there is one relatively new innovation that offers me a great deal of comfort as a soon-to-be patient. It's the ICU Rapid Response Team, now a standard feature in most hospitals. On-call twenty-four hours a day, this mobile "SWAT team" covers the entire hospital, scouting out high-risk or deteriorating patients. If they are alerted quickly to a patient in need and can get there during the crucial "golden hour," as it is called in the scientific literature, treatment is most effective. An ICU nurse is the first responder to arrive and assess the situation. Then, in consultation with a physician and other members of the team, the nurse administers oxygen, fluids, takes blood work, arranges for X-rays, and starts medications. My friend Stephanie, who's on the team, jokingly calls it the "ICU Roadshow." Another friend who's on the team, Janet, says, "it allows us to light a fire under the situation to get things moving along faster." What it does is bring the ICU to patients so that they might not need to come to the ICU. In a way, the Rapid Response Team is like a "virtual ICU" because it's about the people and their expertise, not the place or its equipment. The ICU is a way of doing things.

I have seen the results of the Rapid Response Team and have read the reports: they are catching problems early, preventing mishaps, saving lives, and reducing ICU admissions. What's comforting to me to know as a patient is that anyone – doctor, nurse, patient, family member – can call on them. I plan to keep their phone number close at hand in case I get into trouble post-operatively.

Something else has changed and it's not just at Toronto General Hospital, though TGH has been leading the way. It's the adoption of a corporate philosophy called "patient-centred care" that espouses "respect for patients and their values, beliefs, and concerns . . . and the promotion of physical comfort and emotional and spiritual health . . ." These ideas seemed a "no-brainer" to us nurses when it was first introduced a few years ago. *Wasn't our care already all about the patient?* We were there to meet patients' needs – it's could be the definition of nursing. That's why we chose this profession in the first place – to serve patients. Nursing care *is* patient care. To us, these terms are interchangeable. "Patients R Us" is like "Toys R Us." Would you ask a dentist to be more "teeth-centred?" Yet, the reality was that we often fell short, and we knew it. We've been pulled in too many other directions as we've tried to meet doctors' demands, perform housekeeping, secretarial, and administrative duties, and, of course, all the "hunting and gathering" of equipment and supplies, tending to machines, completing paperwork, and charting on computers – all activities that dragoon us away from patients. Not to mention our own personal failings in trying to meet patient needs.

I will never forget the horrific experience of one nurse who was a patient. Her book, *Bed Number Ten,* had a huge impact on me as a young nurse. Nurse Sue Baier's harrowing account of the cruel and indifferent treatment she received at the hands of hospital staff made me vow to never become one of those callous nurses like the ones who cared for her. Rendered paralyzed by Guillain-Barré syndrome, a rare neurological disorder, Nurse Baier was in the ICU for months and endured unspeakably insensitive, at times cruel, treatment by the staff. I hate to think that there might still be places where patients experience such inhumane treatment, but it's possible.

However, I sense a sea change taking place in the delivery of patient care. Sincere and real efforts are being made to transform the hospital culture into a kinder, friendlier place. These days, patients themselves have a much greater awareness of their right to courteous and respectful care and I hope they will not tolerate any less. Patient affairs departments are there to listen to families' concerns and to step in to mediate conflicts when necessary. Hospitals are making efforts to raise awareness among all staff to improve our communication skills and to be more attuned to patients' needs. We may still fall short at times, but progress is definitely being made. Well, I guess I'll soon find out for myself, won't I?

It's a long and circuitous route to get to the Medical-Surgical ICU where I work, high up on the tenth floor. After the stark, ground-floor entrance hall with its hand-sanitizing stations and the lobby with its potted plastic plants, vinyl chairs and benches bolted to the floor, and rows of philanthropists' bronze busts and donor plaques, you go past a bank of fast-food outlets (communal cafeterias long gone) and commercial gift shops (Volunteer Ladies' Auxiliary Gift Shops vanished) and enter a twisty labyrinth of corridors (where patients are sometimes cared for, when the ER is overflowing, thus the moniker "hallway nursing"). You pass gleaming laboratories and procedure rooms and whiz by "quiet" rooms (a misnomer if there ever was one as they're more like "disquiet" rooms, where patients go to wait and worry) and multifaith worship spaces. Down a sloping hallway past the ICU Reception Area (name changed from "Waiting Room," presumably to take peoples' minds off what they're *really* doing there; it's more of a "Limbo Lounge"), then enter the heavy steel doors and, voilà, the Medical-Surgical ICU, my home away from home.

But tonight I've chosen a different route: I'm taking the stairs. I have to see if I can do it. *Maybe I don't need this surgery after all . . .*

One ... two ... three steps ... A crushing tightness clamps down on my chest. Stopped in my tracks, crouched down on the bottom step, I try to catch my breath.

Out of the corner of my eye, I see inside-out vinyl gloves flung on the stairwell floor right next to what looks like a dried pool of blood but I'm hoping is an old coffee spill. *This place is disgusting! I've seen cleaners swish the filth around in buckets of grey water, push it from one side of the room to the other ... splattered cardiac electrodes, the stinky, soggy blood pressure cuffs ...*

I take the elevator to the tenth floor.

Progress is probably being made in the way nurses work on the wards these days, but years ago, when I was starting out as a new nurse, I was on a general medicine floor and it felt like a brutal reality shock after my protected life as a student. My initiation period was rough. The staff were unfriendly and the workload gruelling. I was constantly thrown into situations I couldn't cope with. There was no one to ask questions about things I was unsure of. I was always running, trying to catch up, constantly frustrated and plagued with the feeling that I was supposed to be somewhere other than where I was, doing something other than what I was doing. It was lonely because there was no teamwork whatsoever, nor any of that "multidisciplinary collaboration" that they promised in school. It was the doctors' world, and nurses were either subordinate, peripheral, or invisible altogether. We were expected to be quiet and just follow orders. Empowered by my enlightened, progressive university education, I had a different vision of how things should be. Though I believed I had more to contribute, I didn't have the courage to speak up and be a maverick. I had no choice but to stick it out because I needed the salary. It was either "sink or swim," so I dogpaddled frantically for almost two years.

Then, when an opportunity came up to study critical care, I didn't know what the ICU entailed, or if I had the right stuff to take it on, or even if the working conditions would be any better, but I took a chance. I did and they were.

I found a lot to love in the ICU. Here, my ideals about nursing could actually be put into practice; the conditions were in place to actually provide patient-centred care – it wasn't a distant dream. Here, my contribution was respected and I could work as equals with the other members of the care team. In fact, our slogan is "Every voice is valued." In the ICU, teamwork is essential because you have to depend on one another; you couldn't do this work alone and you have to be able to count on knowing that whatever comes through the door, we'll deal with it together.

For me personally, the best part was my good fortune to fall in with a group of nurses dubbed "Laura's Line." They soon became mentors and colleagues and now, even though most of them have moved on from the ICU, remain close friends.

For almost thirty years, the ICU has been my home. I know the place, its routines, and all the players. Even so, I try never to lose sight of how unsettling, disturbing – at times terrifying – it is to patients and families, especially when encountering it for the first time. When I bring visitors to their loved one, they stare in dis-belief, hardly recognizing the person, unconscious, entangled in wires and tubes, attached to hulking, noisy machines. One mother insisted I'd brought her to the wrong patient. "This is not my daughter." She stared at the pale, puffy stranger in the bed. I stood at her side while she absorbed the fact that it was.

The ICU is hard-core even for nurses. When it suddenly dawns on you what you're taking on, it's daunting – or should be. I'll never forget the look of utter amazement and discombobulation on one newbie's face as she looked around and pronounced the place "phantasmagorical." She was a Trekkie and nailed it: "They say space is the final frontier, but I think it's here." She was trembling with excitement and fear at the prospect of working here. Laura, the eponymous leader of "Laura's Line," and a buddy of mine, came over to help bring down her stress level a notch or two.

"Relax. It's only machines." Laura gave the ventilator a little kick. "Just keep in mind that that's a person in the bed and it's all about hands-on care, you'll be okay." At that moment, a high-pitched alarm went off. Laura glanced at the monitor and smoothed the patient's covers. "See, it's just an artifact. When an alarm goes off it doesn't necessarily mean something is wrong, only that something *could* be wrong. Your job is to know the difference."

Laura herself could detect a problem long before any machine. To her, the truth was with the patient.

In the ICU, "vital signs" has a different meaning. On the floor, they are taken once a shift; here, they are noted moment by moment. You have to have a solid grasp of normal before you can recognize abnormal. Further, you have to know what normal is for your patient, like a "personal best." Take blood pressure, for example. Before I came to the ICU, I thought of BP as a routine task or something measured once a year at an annual checkup (for those who had them). Very quickly you realize that in the ICU, blood pressure is a big deal. Your patient's blood pressure is always on your mind. We monitor it continuously by a line in the patient's artery and are concerned not only about the systolic and diastolic pressures but a calculated ratio of the two, called the mean arterial pressure (MAP). It reflects the perfusion of the vital organs, but I tend to think of MAP as the force that propels life forward. To me, MAP is that poetic.

Heartbeats are given equally close attention as we examine them in second intervals, measure parts of them in milliseconds. We are constantly sizing up whether the hearth rhythm is regularly regular, regularly irregular, irregularly regular. The same close attention is given to breathing. Second by second, breath by breath, each is counted and measured, as well as the intervals in between breaths.

Then there's urine! We note the colour, if there is sediment, and the amount, millilitre by millilitre, we tally it hourly, not just allow it to accumulate to the end of the shift. In the ICU, all the elements of life – cells, enzymes, minerals, electrolytes, and microbes – are under scrutiny. Moment by moment, bodies are in the balance – beating, dripping, dropping, ticking, pulsing, and pumping.

Another thing I love about the ICU is that everything about my patient is my business: heartbeats my responsibility to safeguard, each drop of urine my concern. I'll never forget the first time I heard an ICU nurse say, "My pressure's low," and realized she meant her *patient's* blood pressure. "It's like when your child coughs, it's your cough, too," she explained.

A nurse has to earn the privilege to work here – and stay. You have to study hard and keep on top of your game, proving yourself over and over again. The learning curve is steep, especially at first. For me, the technical skills came slowly and acquiring the mandatory knowledge and critical thinking took even longer. As for the emotional fortitude – well, I'm still working on that.

"Why are you still there?" friends often ask. "Isn't it time to move on to bigger and better things?"

Like what? I wonder. What could top this? I've found my place. To me, what happens at the bedside is the most interesting and important thing – and in the ICU, I couldn't get any closer to the bedside. Besides, why would I leave when I haven't mastered it? I'm still trying to get it right.

"You're just here for the stories," some nurses tease me.

I'll admit it – I'm an adrenalin junkie, getting high on the drama and action and grappling with the various complicated ethical dilemmas, but my real fix is stories. I never tire of being let into my patients' lives. I'm insatiably curious about the multitude of challenges that people face and the infinite ways they respond to them.

As fascinating as it all is, I rarely let outsiders into my world. I don't tell my friends or family much. When I do, they either don't get it or it makes them worry about themselves – or me. Then I have to reassure them that I'm okay. *This is what I've chosen, what I love to do.* I have never nursed sick children, worked in disaster zones in the aftermath of earthquakes or floods. I've never taken care of trauma victims, women in labour, or babies, only critically ill adults. Violence, cruelty, trauma, abuse are harder for me to compute, but illness, disease, and existential suffering make more sense to me.

Our patients have complicated metabolic diseases, overwhelming infections, or rare auto-immune disorders; many have undergone major thoracic (chest) or abdominal surgeries or organ transplants. Some have multiple organ failure; few have only one thing wrong with them. Many, but by no means all, are elderly. In all cases, outcomes are uncertain. But there is one thing there's no getting around: our patients suffer. We do our best to ameliorate their discomfort, but there's no denying it. At times, it's hard to tell the difference between the suffering caused by the illness and that caused by the treatments. More than anything, there are always more questions than answers, way more problems than solutions. "We're like *csi* detectives," one nurse said, "always gathering evidence, building a case, trying to solve puzzles."

After the mystery is "solved," more or less, our patients move on to a step-down unit or a medical or surgical floor. When they eventually go home, they don't usually stay in touch, but a few do. One grateful patient took the time to write to us recently:

You first met me as a very sick patient on the verge of death.
Tomorrow I will be transferred to the rehab centre. You kept
me alive to make this possible. I am so grateful for your skills
and care. My two grandchildren will now see much more of
grandma. Bill and I will continue to grow old together and
enjoy ourselves. Thank you from the bottom of my heart . . .

It's lovely to hear from them, but those aren't the ones we get to
know as we do the ones that end up with complications, whose
paths are rocky and turbulent. They loom larger in our psyches.
In other parts of the hospital there are faster turnarounds, even
"miraculous" recoveries, but here, triumphs are hard-won and
tenuous; progress more fragile, usually partial and imperfect. It's
more of a slogging away, a day at a time, two steps forward, one
back, or one step forward and two back. *Down seven, up eight.*

And yes, over the years, I have seen many deaths. I once had an
argument with an administrator who designed a poster to represent our ICU. She chose a photograph of a sunset and a tree, the light
glinting through the leaves at sunset. It sends the wrong image, I
insisted. People come here to fight. The pastoral beauty of nature
is not what inspires them here; they want cutting-edge science and
sophisticated technology. This is not a hospice or a place to die – at
least not at first. We admit a patient to the ICU because we believe
we can make them better – at least it starts off that way.

But not everything can be fixed and death can't always be
"cheated," as we like to believe. Those of us who've worked here
for any length of time have seen too much of the other side of
things – or maybe that's just what we remember best.

"Do the math," said a friend, another old-timer who's worked
here twenty-five-plus years like me. "We've witnessed the equivalent of the death of an entire town."

True, but it's not the numbers that stay with you, it's the stories. For most of us, it's not the death, but the way many people die, spending their last days cared for by strangers, in this alien environment, tethered to machines, chrome, and plastic.

Most of our patients do get better — we do have many success stories, for example, organ transplants. Rarely an easy course, but when all goes well, it is thrilling to meet the recipients, walking and talking, weeks later. Through the selflessness of a family who has just received the worst news of their lives, or the generosity of a family member or friend, the gift of lungs, kidney, pancreas, heart, or liver can save lives. No one who does this work can fail to be in awe when that happens.

Tonight, the hustle and bustle at change of shift is at a fever-pitch. There are some *sick* people. I catch fragments of conversations as I pass by the rooms.

". . . forty-two-year-old female, idiopathic pulmonary hypertension . . . satting only 71 per cent on 100 per cent oxygen . . . awaiting lung transplant . . . top of the organ list."

". . . twenty-eight-year-old male, found at a bar . . . overdosed on Ecstacy . . . unconscious, tachycardic . . . no urine output . . . kidneys shut down — not even bladder sweat . . . dialysis to be started shortly . . . can't locate family."

". . . Rapid Response Team bringing patient from the floor . . . eighty-two-year-old, unconscious, in respiratory failure . . . needs intubation . . . family is too distraught right now for a discussion, but we need to make some decisions about the plan of care . . ."

I adjust my ears to the ICU background music, a playlist of dings, dongs, chirps, buzzes, and beeps going off at random intervals from patient rooms. I never noticed it before but this place is noisy. Heavy doors bang open and close, rushed footsteps, loud voices

– even peels of laughter and excited chatter at the nursing station. As for tonight's vintage bouquet? I sniff the air and catch a whiff of a fresh upper gastro-intestinal bleed, the sweet-sour undertones of a brewing pseudomonas infection, and do I detect a frisson of melena – the distinctive smell of the end result of that GI blood passing through the "lower" end?

The housekeeping staff are cleaning rooms and restocking cupboards as they finish their shifts. Cindy, Comfort, and Eunice speak in a mélange of Chinese-, African-, and Jamaican-inflected English. They wave or call out *hey* as I make my way to the nursing station. There, David, a tall, elegant man, a patient care assistant, greets me in his courtly manner.

"Good evening, young lady." He makes a deep bow. "I'm pleased to see you've decided to grace us with your presence on this lovely evening."

The twenty-four ICU beds are full, I see, as I make my way around the spacious, rectangular-shaped unit to check the assignment board to find out the name of my patient. Most of our patients are so ill and unstable that they require one-to-one nursing care. In some cases, two nurses are needed to care for one patient.

For years, I've had a mystical belief that I always get the patient I need. (Whether my patients get the nurse they need is another story, and whether as a patient I'll get the nurses I need remains to be seen.) For example, if my energy is flagging and I'm assigned a very sick patient, it's a sign to dig down deep and rise to the occasion. A "quiet," or stable, patient is a cue to make myself available to other nurses who need my assistance. I become the nurse I need to be. Tonight, with my own worries on my mind, all I'm hoping is to be a Good-Enough Nurse who can get my patient safely through the night. One bed full of suffering is all I can cope with right now.

Ramona, the day nurse, is standing outside the patient's room waiting for me. She's been here all day and is eager to hand over so she can go home. She launches straight into her report on our patient, a sixty-six-year-old First Nations man admitted to the hospital three weeks ago for abdominal surgery for a bowel obstruction who then developed pneumonia and respiratory failure.

"Mr. Beausoleil — he likes to be called George — awake and alert, oriented to person, place, and time. Restless and confused at times. I gave him Haldol 2.5 milligrams IV twice today. Tolerated well, but we're trying to minimize sedation because we're hoping to extubate him in the morning. On pressure support of five, oxygen at 35 per cent . . . if he doesn't fly he'll need a trach. Gets tachypneic with anxiety — his resp. rate goes up to fifty or so. Cardiac status stable . . . normal sinus rhythm with no ectopics; blood pressure stable. Line-wise, he's got a subclavian triple lumen catheter — site was changed two days ago — with normal saline to keep the vein open . . . magnesium was low so I topped him up with two grams. On insulin nomogram . . . last blood sugar 10.2 millimoles."

I'm used to this barrage of rat-tat-tat facts coming at me in rapid-fire bullets. I let it wash over me as I mentally highlight key points, what needs clarification, and what questions remain, like this one:

"Any family?" What I need to know is anyone hovering out in the waiting room, anxious to come in. I want to know who cares about this man in his life outside the hospital, other than me, tonight for twelve hours, for whom it is my job to do so?

"Oops, forgot about that. No one came to visit. His wife died a few years ago. There's a daughter in Vancouver, but she didn't call today."

A sad but all-too-common situation.

But what's uppermost on my mind is this question: Would I have Ramona as my nurse? Yes. She's a just-the-facts-ma'am kind of nurse, but I probably wouldn't die on her watch.

Before going in, I glance through the window at a frail, elderly man, his arms tied down in restraints. The sedation Ramona gave him has kicked in so I wonder if he still needs them. Most of us do all we can to avoid physical restraints, but if patients are at risk for pulling out their lines or endotracheal tubes (breathing tubes), we have no choice. Some patients can't be soothed with words, touch, or even drugs. A restless patient can be more challenging to care for than a combative or even violent one; it's a persistent, gnawing need that's never quelled or satisfied. You do your best to keep your cool, but we've all had moments of impatience. One time I was so rattled by a patient's agitated state that I caught myself shouting, "Calm down!" as if calmness could be commanded. Justine, my pal from Laura's Line, used to call it "going nurse!" instead of "going postal!"

Doctors don't get this. If they pass by a patient's room and happen to see the patient in a moment of rest, that's their snapshot impression. Even if the patient is agitated, it doesn't affect them like it does us. They aren't required to be as up close and personal for such extended periods of time as we are. They can keep a remove of time, space, and often emotion, too. One thing that helps me is keeping in mind the motto of the "Dog Whisperer." Cesar Millan advises people to stay "calm and assertive" when dealing with unruly canines. (Though I don't have a dog, I watch the show and aspire to be a "Patient Whisperer" by putting into practice Cesar's advice about "fulfilling the other's needs" and helping them attain "balanced energy.")

After introducing myself to my patient, I loosen the restraints on his arms and then begin my head-to-toe assessment, starting with his level of consciousness. Though he's awake and alert, he can't speak because of the breathing tube in his mouth, which, by necessity, passes through his vocal cords.

"How are you doing tonight?" I ask and he motions for a clipboard to write on.

I wish to god i felt better.

"Anything in particular bothering you?"

He shakes his head and sets aside the clipboard beside him on the bed.

"Just being here, huh?" He nods. "Do you know what day is it?" I ask and he shrugs his shoulder to indicate he hasn't a clue, so I tell him. It's easy to lose track of time here, cut off from the world. When I wake up in the morning or especially in the middle of the night, the first thing I do is check my watch or clock.

When I tell George it's Saturday night, June 30, he moves his legs and arms like he's out dancing on the town. He reaches for the clipboard again.

Want to get away from here for a day or two. Come with me?

"Love to." I strip off a vinyl glove so that I can touch his hand, skin to skin. This can be a hazardous practice, possibly exposing me to infectious bodily fluids, but sometimes I take the risk. George points to the eagle tattoo on his shoulders and tries to tell me something but falls back against the pillow, too weak to get the words out clearly.

"Maybe later you'll be able to tell me?" I ask and he nods.

The night wears on. As I monitor his heart, record his hourly vital signs, suction his lungs, give him his meds, and change his chest tube dressing, I can't help but think about my own heart, vital signs, lungs, the meds that will be given to me, and the wound I'll have. *I'll be in the hands of strangers, just like George.*

Tonight, some of my buddies are on duty. There's Jasna, who is in charge of the ICU this shift, making her rounds, checking on the patients and the nurses, too. Stephanie is in her patient's room, the curtains closed. I don't expect to see much of Janet. It's her turn on the Rapid Response Team. She'll be making her rounds, following up on patients who've recently been discharged from the ICU to the step-down unit or answering calls for help from the floor, always on the alert for patients in trouble or, as Janet puts it, "people making mischief in the night."

She's explained to me how it works. "Anyone can page us, a nurse, doctor, or even a family member. We go there, size up the situation, figure out if it's a hot A – a patient who needs to come to the ICU ASAP! A B is a worrisome or iffy patient. It's a 'heads-up' that this patient needs to be followed closely. We try to fix them on the floor so they won't have to come to the ICU. A good save like that is an amazing feeling! Then there's a C, which is a consult about someone who's stable but not looking good. It's someone that someone is worried about. You've got to trust your gut and use your noggin. Sometimes we just offer advice or teaching, nurse to nurse, say, about pain management or symptom control. Some of those nurses on the floor are very experienced. But they don't have time to help the rookies – so that's what we're there for."

To me, this advanced role sounds daunting, but Janet is quick to explain that they don't do anything without running it by the doctor first and getting an order, and that all decisions are made together. "We're the eyes and ears, right at the scene, telling them what we see and what we think." She's serious and emphatic about that, but in a moment the old twinkle in her eye reappears. "But

what usually happens is we've figured out the problem and have
a pretty good idea what needs to be done by the time we've called
the doctor."

To be chosen to become a member of the Rapid Response Team,
you have to be an experienced nurse, undergo additional education,
and have proven yourself capable of this advancement. I haven't
taken it on myself but hope to one day.

I look over at my partner for the night, Simone. She has been
an ICU nurse only a few months, a nurse less than a year. There
aren't many nurses who are capable of working in the ICU so soon
after graduating from nursing school, but Simone might be one
who is. What she lacks in experience, she more than makes up
for in book smarts and an eagerness to learn. At first glance it
would seem unwise, even unsafe, to pair an inexperienced nurse
with a complex and unstable lung transplant patient, but new
nurses will never come into their own if they aren't given challenges, especially under the watchful eye of a well-seasoned
(sounds like a roast turkey) veteran. That's where I come in. It's
how I learned.

I'd been hoping to coast tonight, but I'll need to keep my radar
out to help Simone if she needs it. So far, she doesn't seem worried, not the least bit daunted, but I have a feeling she should be.

It's less than an hour into the shift and Simone is in over her
head. I go over to help, staying mere steps from my own patient and
well within earshot of him and his monitor alarms. At first Simone
balks at what she sees as my interference, saying she can manage
on her own, but quickly softens when she realizes that I'm here to
help, not to criticize. She's clearly overwhelmed, glancing from the
monitor, to her patient, to the countertop cluttered with meds due
to be administered, not sure where to start first. Her patient's
ventilator alarm keeps going off and she silences it without

checking the reason. The family has been calling in repeatedly
from the waiting room, asking to come in, and she is flustered,
snapping at them over the phone, *Not now.* I go over and suction her
patient's lungs and give him an extra boost of oxygen. I change the
chest tube drainage system that has filled up with bloody drainage
and then start sorting out the "spaghetti," the tangled-up, inter-
twined iv lines. Her patient has a fever and a high white count and
needs blood cultures, so I do that. Together, we check and double-
check, then co-sign for two units of blood, and I prime blood
tubing, then prepare extra drips of iv Levophed and epinephrine.
These powerful meds are running in each of the iv ports and cannot
be put on hold while the blood runs in.

"After the antibiotic runs in, a port will be freed up to hang the
blood," she reasons.

"But you have other meds due and your hemoglobin is only sixty.
Your patient needs the blood now. It can't wait. You'll have to start
a peripheral iv and let the doctor know we need a new central line.
This one may be a source of infection."

"I'm not good at them," she admits, eyeballing her patient's arm.

Veins are one of my specialties. The plump ones look juicy, but
I don't fall for that easy temptation. I prefer the ones you can feel
rather than see. First, I send her on a scavenger hunt to collect
what's needed. It's like a *mis en place* before preparing a complicated French recipe: if you assemble the angiocath, tourniquet,
alcohol wipes, and prime the iv tubing before starting to "cook,"
you won't be scrambling and will calmly nab that vein. It doesn't
seem that long ago that I was bumbling around, coming into a
patient's room, forgetting to bring something, going out to get it,
coming back in again, running around in circles. "Have you started
many ivs before?" I ask Simone when everything is ready.

"Yeah, but only on the simulator models at university."

Ahh, this is the new nursing education, a more *in vitro* process than *in vivo*. What Simone means is that she learned to take a pulse, auscultate lungs, and perform other skills on high-fidelity dummies made of plastic, rubber, silicone, and computer chips. They even mimic human responses like crying out in pain or expressing distress. What they don't mimic is the disruptions, distractions, interruptions, fatigue, and simultaneous multi-tasking of real-life nursing.

Way back in the day when I was a nursing student, we prac-tised our skills on one another before working with patients under the close supervision of an experienced nurse. It was the old-fashioned training or apprentice system. We took blood pres-sures, drew blood, and once, we even inserted naso-gastic tubes into one another. (This is a catheter that goes into the nose, down the throat, and into the stomach, used to drain fluids, deflate air, or give medications.) It was unpleasant, but every single time I've done that procedure to a patient, I remember how it feels. You can't get that from an electronic dummy, just as you can't pilot a plane after playing a flight simulation game. Something is lost. It fosters the kind of detachment I saw in one young nurse. She sat outside the room, staring at a computer screen, glancing now and then at the patient's cardiac monitor and ventilator screen. Later, standing at the bedside, she pushed buttons and recorded data from the machines. She didn't touch or speak to the patient, nor make eye contact. It was nursing by numbers with no connection to the person in the bed.

But how to teach empathy? Compassion may be innate in some, but not in most of us. The skills of face-to-face interaction may be challenging to the "net generation," or "millenials," since many are more familiar with online relationships, electronic connec-tions, and virtual realities than one-on-one, real-life ones. But the new nurses teach me a lot, too, and I love being around them with their verve, idealism, and self-confidence. Their ease in learning new things and their refusal to compromise their personal lives for their careers is inspiring. They've all had a chuckle at our old-school ways, like our resistance to new computer programs or when the automated medication dispensing machines were introduced. They were patient with us, holding our hands until we were up to speed. They want to learn from us, but unfortunately not enough of us are willing to work closely with them and impart what we know, thus the need for laboratory models to practise on. Paradoxically, you have to be young to do this work but old enough to do it right (though "old" or "young" in this context has nothing to do with age).

Under my guidance, Simone gets the IV in and looks pleased with herself. Everything is under control for now, so I suggest it's time to bring the family in, but she doesn't feel ready because the room is still messy and she wants to tidy it up.

"None of that matters," I tell her. "They've waited long enough. Bring them in."

I'm not always so helpful — or bossy — but I feel a new urgency to pass the torch.

Nathan, our ward clerk, dims the hallway lights, an encouraging sign that nudges the night along.

My patient appears to be sleeping, but it can be hard to tell; I've cared for patients who looked like they were in a deep sleep but tell me in the morning they didn't have a moment of rest. His vital signs are stable and I make sure his monitor alarms are on. "Listen out for a minute, would you?" I call out to Simone to let her know I'll be stepping away from the bedside for a moment. It means *Stay tuned to my patient's alarms, extend your radar to cover my patient, too. You are responsible for both of them.* There isn't a crisis every minute, but in the ICU, there's a constant expectation of close observation and quick response should a problem arise and so our patients can't be left alone, not even for a minute to step out to for supplies or a bathroom run. I alert Jasna, too, so there'll be a nurse for the nurse as well as one for the patient.

I take a stroll around the ICU, pausing outside each patient's door to peer inside, to watch not the patients but the nurses.

There's Wendy, who brings a sense of order and peace as she chats quietly with her patient and at the same time checks his chest tube drainage and urine output. He's a nineteen-year-old boy with cystic fibrosis, two days post-op lung transplant, just extubated and experiencing what it feels like to breathe easily for the first time in his life.

Diana has her arm protectively around her patient's wife as she explains something about her husband's condition, in her excitable yet comforting way, as they stand outside his door.

Holly is caring for her patient behind a closed curtain, talking to him softly.

Kelly is on the phone calling all over the hospital, hunting down a drug her patient needs right away. There's no time to waste; waiting until the morning might be too late.

I can hear Jason (who's Chinese) speaking Tamil to his Sri Lankan patient. (Welcome to Toronto!) He reads from a "cheat sheet" prepared by the family for us to use. "Naan ippoothu unkalai marupakkam thiruppa paakiren. Iruma seiya paakum," he says to let her know he's going to turn her and that it might make her cough.

And anyone who is still under the misconception that men aren't as nurturing as women should hear "Big John," a manly, strapping, huntin' and fishin' kinda guy, speaking to his patient, a thirty-nine-year-old woman with breast cancer and now pneumonia: "It's 11:30 at night. David is here to help me to turn you to the other side and I'll give your sore back a rub. You're doing great, darlin'. I'll suction the secretions out of your lungs first. Easy does it. You're safe. I'm right here with you — not going anywhere."

I move on to Stephanie's room and I can see in an instant that her patient is sick — the sickest patient in the ICU tonight. I don't know if Stephanie got the patient she needed, but her patient — a twenty-three-year-old woman in septic shock — surely got the nurse she needed. If it's possible to do so, Stephanie will pull her through.

There are many such A-listers who work here, including Edna, Allyson, Grace, Connie, Murry, Kate, Lesley, Marcia. From whatever angle you observe them, whatever moment you chose, they are reliably doing something that makes the situation better and safer. Oh, there are a few D-listers, too, but we keep them in check. It's always like that: some extraordinary professionals, a tiny group of stragglers, and the majority of us in the satisfactory middle. But nurses are the wild card. You don't know what you are going to get. I remember how one patient put it. "How's it going?" I asked at the start of my shift.

"Depends on the day."

"How about this day?"

"Depends on the nurse."

I get this. The nurse can make all the difference for good or bad.

The wife of one of my patients was fond of me, at least at first. I think it was because of my optimism. Well, in the morning I felt that way, but by the late afternoon her husband's condition had worsened dramatically and we were working hard to keep him alive. I felt less certain that he would make it, and had not as much time and energy to devote to reassuring and comforting her because I had to stay focused on his care. I watched her mood plummet. "I'm not feeling as good about things as I felt this morning," she said, searching my eyes for my faith so that she could be buoyed up again. But frankly, I didn't have as much to give. I tried to fake it but I could see I'd lost her trust. The next day, she requested a different nurse.

Privately, we ask ourselves, "Would you want this nurse to take care of you?" (The more telling question is, which nurse *wouldn't* you want?) Yes, I'd have Simone, as long as an experienced nurse is also there to back her up and watch my back at the same time. Problem is, not enough of us "golden oldies" are willing to light the way for the newbies. We say we're busy or too burnt out. *I'm nursing the patient, do I have to nurse the nurse, too?* they ask. I say, Yes, you do. How else will we pass on the collective wisdom of this profession and sustain it? Too many of us are complaining and acting dissatisfied but not expressing what we treasure or why we've stayed, other than it pays the bills.

I see I've gone from worrying which patient I'll get to which nurse I'll get. Does my karmic theory have a corollary – will I get the nurse I need? I'll soon find out.

It's two o'clock in the morning and Simone comes over to sit beside me at the desk outside our patients' room, a post from where we can still observe them and their machines. She looks tired. Because we always work in pairs, on a buddy system, when it is safe to do so we cover each other's patients and spell each other off so we can take breaks during the night, sometimes even naps.

"If you need to lie down for a while, I can cover your patient for you," I offer, but she says she's too keyed up to take a break.

"I don't feel well. I should have called in sick," she says, looking more stressed and fatigued than ill. "Nights suck, don't they?" she says with a sigh. "Do you ever get used to them?"

"Not really. I still find them hard." There's no getting around it – night shift is hard. On the upside, it allows you to escape the hubbub and politics that goes on during the day, but you feel cut off from the rest of the team, not to mention your family, friends, and normal life, which, for most people takes place during the day. Working all night is unfathomable to non-nurse friends. You feel embarrassed to admit you're working Saturday night. They pity you, and you feel a bit sorry for yourself, too.

I don't work nearly as many nights now as I used to, but there was a time when I worked so many nights that three o'clock in the morning felt exactly the same as three o'clock in the afternoon. I used to dread coming in, having to tear myself away from friends or family. For years I worked my share of nights (the union decreeing that we split our shifts equally between nights and days), always fighting off an exaggerated feeling of loneliness and isolation from the rest of the world during those dark hours. Most nights I managed to attain the minimal wakefulness required to be safe. Over the years, I've learned to make peace with working the night shift, which isn't to say that at the age of almost-fifty it isn't difficult, but then again, it was back in my twenties, too. It's never felt normal or healthy to work at night and sleep all day. But patients need nursing care around the clock, so the night shift is here to stay.

George is now awake and indicates that he's uncomfortable, so I call for David to help me reposition him. Then I draw the curtains and give my patient a bath, not as much for hygiene as for relaxation. Washing him as I do, soaping his armpits, rubbing his back, massaging his fingers one by one, cleaning his legs, pulling back the foreskin, wiping the folds around the scrotum, actions that in any other context would be sexual. These professional intimacies are decidedly not, but they aren't strictly clinical either. We each find our own ways to deal with any discomfiting thoughts that come up in these situations of vulnerability, shame, or embarrassment –

at times, our own.

Some nurses seem disinterested or disappointed by these seemingly mundane aspects of patient care. "I like everything about nursing," one told me, "except actual patient care." Perhaps they believe that their university education qualifies them to do "better" things and that such "menial" work is beneath them. It's a class, even a caste, prejudice. Their academic, theoretical education does not adequately prepare them for the shocking realities of the hospital. Patient care seems to have a low priority on the nursing curricula in universities, not accorded the importance it deserves. *Knowledge workers* is the new phrase to describe our role, and while it's a true description, there is also body work and, for many of us, a spiritual component, too. But many new nurses tell me they don't plan to stay at the bedside for long. For many, patient care is merely a stepping stone in their career path before moving on to teaching, research, administration, management, or graduate school. Years ago, I felt as they do, and wanted to move on to "better things," but that was before I saw how nurses heal people with their hands and minds, with their actions and their words. Soon, I discovered that for me, there is no work more meaningful and satisfying than patient care.

George is still uncomfortable. I ask if he's in pain. He nods but can't say where or how much, but I don't need evidence. He has plenty of reasons to have physical pain, and mental anguish, too. We know a lot now about ICU delirium, a syndrome that can exhibit as confusion, hallucinations, delusions, nightmares, and an altered sleep-awake cycle. It affects up to 80 per cent of ICU patients and a large number of hospitalized patients, particularly the elderly. It can even cause post-traumatic stress syndrome, with long-term flashbacks, bad memories, and nightmares, all from an ICU stay. We use sedation and antipsychotic medications to treat this problem, which, as a nurse, you have to be on the lookout for its signs and symptoms at all times.

I draw up a dose of sedation and inject it into his IV, a central line that goes into a large vein that leads directly into his heart. *What a leap of faith it takes to allow someone to inject a drug into your veins!* Just before nodding off, he mouths, "Thank you" around the ETT tube, a message that's easy to decipher. Most of us have learned to read lips — eyebrows, foreheads, shoulders, fingers, and toes, too.

If my patient gets a good sleep, in the morning when he's extubated, he'll do better. But so far, he's not having a restful night, sleeping on and off, mostly off.

I stand outside my doorway for a moment and call out to Stephanie as she flies past my room, but she's so focused on what she's doing she doesn't even stop to say hello. "Busy patient?" I call out, but I can hear and see the answer for myself by peeking into her patient's room. The overhead lights are on. The noisy high-speed oscillator ventilator is going full blast, pounding hundreds of tiny breaths into her patient's lungs per minute. The counter is lined with syringes of medications and there's a stack of IV pumps attached to her patient. Classic signs of a *busy patient*. That phrase is so ICU. Once, I told a friend I had a busy patient and he thought I meant a "workaholic," talking on a cellphone, using a computer, doing business from his hospital bed! No, *busy patient* means a busy nurse.

I return to my patient's room and see that he is wide awake, and restless, pulling at his ventilator tubing and trying to tell me something. He motions for the clipboard.

Are you back tonight?

I know what lies behind that question. He's come to trust me and now he's going to have to trust someone new. Patients often ask why they get a different nurse every day. They've gotten used to the quirks of Nurses Dawn, Mercedes, and Hasmina and now it's May-Ling, Trey, and Scott? Each nurse is so different in personality, style, tone, tempo, and energy – and I know patients feel it.

The way we make up the patient assignment must seem so random and arbitrary to them, but there's actually logic to it, but it's hard to crack the code. Though we want to provide consistency of staff to achieve a "continuity of care," the reality is that with the vagaries of hundreds of work, family, and school schedules, along with nurses' varying skill sets and all the complicated personality alchemies, it is difficult to do so.

On top of that, we try to take into consideration certain sensitive situations, like not assigning a nurse who's had a recent death in the family to care for a dying patient. Nurses themselves sometimes request assignment changes because, as one exasperated nurse put it, "my patient was driving me friggin' crazy" or as another said, visibly disappointed in herself, "I tried my best, but I just wasn't gelling with the family." We keep a secret[*] book, not officially acknowledged by management, stashed in a drawer at the front desk in which we record the challenging or "difficult," long-term patients so as to not overburden any individuals. We would like to be above such personal failings, but most of us aren't – though that's no excuse. It would be nice to offer bespoke care; nursing is neither a one-size-fits-all enterprise nor a one-way interaction. But the expectation that we will be able to care for any and every patient at any time doesn't jibe with reality.

"No, I won't be back," I tell my patient gently. "This is my last shift for a while."

---

[*]   Not anymore!

His disappointment is a compliment. He wants me back. He motions for the clipboard:

> When you go Home can you take me
> with you Please

Desperation, so politely put.

There's something else he wants to tell me. Through gestures, mouthing words, and pantomime, he manages to tell me the story of the eagle tattoo on his shoulder . . . why the wings face backward. "The eagle has my back," he tells me and gives a toothless grin around the plastic tube in his mouth.

That's what he was trying to tell me earlier. I nod in understanding.

"You are doing so well," I tell him. "We'll get that breathing tube out this morning. You'll be able to talk." I squeeze his hand and he squeezes mine in return.

It's 0500 hours, time to record another set of vital signs and perform my hourly checks.

There's somewhere I need to go, something I need to do. I promise Simone I won't be gone for long and ask Jasna to cover our patients as well. I leave the ICU and take the elevator down to the Cardiovascular ICU. I am looking for Meera, a friend who left Med-Surg for CV because, as she puts it, "it's cleaner" – meaning fewer infections – "and most people get better" – meaning they have (usually) one fixable problem.

"Meera isn't on tonight," the nurse-in-charge tells me but doesn't seem to mind my hanging around at the nursing station. She has no idea I'm here on a reconnaissance mission, spying and checking out the place, wondering which bed I'll be in and which nurses will be taking care of me.

A caravan is making its way down the hall. The patient on the stretcher is motionless, eyes taped shut, flanked on all sides by people pushing poles of IV pumps with green and red lights flash-ing (the reason we call them "Christmas trees").

"Quadruple bypass," the in-charge says as they pass the nursing station. "We took him back to the OR. Bleeding."

"What's going on in there?" I point to a room so crowded I can't even see the patient in the bed.

"Two days post-op heart transplant. They're evacuating a tamponade."

Here's yet another post-op complication. Cardiac tamponade is fluid in the pericardial sac surrounding the heart that impedes blood flow. The ultrasound technologist is guiding the surgeon to place the needle to relieve the pressure.

There's a different vibe here. Even with this crisis, all is calm. In my ICU, it's more chaotic, the rhythm more erratic. We either go full-tilt, non-stop or ride out a steady, slow burn with uneasy lulls. We do more guesswork, try this or that, see what works. We manage problems, but here they fix them.

The ultrasound technologist comes out, wheeling his machine ahead of him.

"Hey, Gary. How're you doing?" I greet him.

"Good," he says cheerfully, "as long as I stay on this side of the bedrails."

As if he knew!

On my way back to the ICU, I run into Janet making her rounds, "checking on my babies," as she says. "Gotta make sure everyone's hunky-dory." We stop to chat. "Are you *bagelling* with us this morn-ing, Tillie?" she asks, rushing away when her beeper goes off.

"I'm in," I call out, though I'm in no mood for the jovial cream cheese chatter.

I've been gone about twenty minutes and it's time to get back to my patient. As I'm rushing through the halls back to the ICU, stopping occasionally to catch my breath, I hear, "Code Blue, Code Blue." I wonder if it was the patient that Janet was on her way to see. The person may need to come to the ICU, I think. *It's not my problem. I'm going home,* I remind myself.

Soon Ramona, the day-shift nurse, arrives back and now our situation is reversed. I know everything about our shared patient and she's starting all over again. I rush through my report and hurry off. George is sleeping so there's no opportunity to say good-bye. I would have liked to be there when he's extubated and hear his voice, but it's time to go. So often it's like this. We get to read only one page in a chapter of a person's life and don't get to hear how the story turns out.

"Thanks for your help, Tilda," Simone calls out. "You were awesome."

Before leaving the ICU, I slip a note under the office door of Denise, our manager, to let her know I'll be off on an extended sick leave, much longer than the two weeks I'd booked off for camp. *Will call to explain.*

I walk out and don't look back.

After most of my friends from Laura's Line left the ICU, I joined a new group: The Bagel Club. There's Janet, a.k.a. the Grand Poo-Bah; Stephanie, a.k.a. Shorty; and Jasna, a.k.a. Jazzy. They call me Tillie. Every second Sunday morning after night shift we go *bagelling.* It's not a legit Yiddish word (though it sounds like it could be), just another of Janet's spoonerisms. Eric Bailis, the owner of St. Urbain's Bagels on Bathurst Street, greets us. "Lose anyone last night?" he always asks, though we never tell him if we did. The place is steamy, fragrant with coffee and hot bagels. It's hopping with regulars who fill brown paper bags with bagels and pastries, then stop by our table to say hi and joke, "Save any lives?" and then seek advice about a skin condition, a knee problem, a mother who has Alzheimer's.

When we first started coming to this suburban Jewish enclave in Thornhill, the Sunday-morning tradition and the friendly but argumentative clientele was a new experience for these friends. I took it as my duty to explain the incessant *kibitzing* and *shmoozing* (gossiping and kidding around), the frequent *kvetching* (whining and complaining), and constant *fressing* and *noshing* (snacking and nibbling). I filled them in on the age-old rivalries between fans of Montreal-style bagels (chewy, dense, slightly sweet) versus Toronto-style (fluffier, heavier, saltier) along with bagel etiquette, such as not toasting a fresh bagel and discouraging ersatz varieties such as sun-dried tomato or chocolate chip. They are amused whenever I recount the corny, nutshell version of Jewish history: "They tried to kill us, we survived, now let's eat!"

"Is this what they learn you in the sin-ee-gogue?" Janet asks. With her baby blue eyes, brilliantly blonde hair (which she comes by naturally, I know she'd want me to add), and mock hillbilly voice, she likes to act like a white trash hick chick but she's actually a sophisticated culture vulture. A huge reader, her taste is classic and high-brow (favourites are Jane Austen and Thomas Hardy), plus she's a world traveller who's been to France, Italy, and Denmark. With her gregarious and playful personality, curvaceous figure, and robust good looks, Janet stands out in any group. She's always bursting with life and has a full-of-beans personality – such fun to be around! – and though she may look cherubic, there is a permanent mischievous twinkle in those baby blues. She sits, sipping a hot chocolate, proudly wearing an oversized T-shirt emblazoned with one of the many charities for which she's the volunteer captain of the medical team. Today it's bright yellow Ride to Conquer Cancer, and with the event, a bike ride from Toronto to Niagara Falls, coming up soon, she's recruiting additional volunteers. I turn it down but can't bring myself to tell her why.

After a shift, we always are dress in our casual, comfy clothes, having thrown our used uniforms into the hospital laundry or brought them home for laundering. (Wearing scrubs outside of work is strictly taboo due to infection control concerns and the unprofessional image it projects, despite the fact that you'll see this infraction around town in grocery stores or coffee shops. All I can say about that is: *Yuck.*)

Jasna sips on a chamomile tea. Her quieter, even-tempered presence is a calming flava to our group. Always dressed down and understated, Jasna is implacable and gentle, though she occasionally gives a sly smile and surprises us with an insightful zinger. Modest to a fault, Jasna seriously contemplated being a no-show at a recent award ceremony in honour of her outstand-ing nursing care.

Then there's Stephanie, a petite, sassy ball of pure energy. She often says she's tired but never looks it or acts it and always gives her all to every patient in her care. She's arguably the best dresser among us in her faded jeans, leather bomber jacket, and kick-ass boots – finds from second-hand clothing shops and bargain base-ments that she sources out as much for economical reasons as environmental ones.

There is so much I admire about these women, but as nurses what I love the most is how they always do what's right for their patients and will fight for them, if necessary.

"Do we have a quorum?" Stephanie starts off, as if it's a formal meeting.

Now that they've finished their bagels, they wipe their hands and reach into their bags for balls of yarn and knitting needles. An hour ago in the hospital, they wielded another type of needle, and their handiwork was patient care. Janet is knitting a soft, custard yellow baby blanket; Jasna, fingerless gloves for driving; and Stephanie, a pair of socks. (She says she only knits socks, claiming she doesn't have patience for the sweater I've been begging her to make me.) Their knitting is the cue to pull out my tools: a pen and paper, but last night before work, in my distracted state, I forgot to throw my notebook into my knapsack. Ever helpful, Jasna flattens open the empty paper bag from the bagels and hands it to me, along with a pen.

"Be careful what you say." Stephanie gives a sideways glance at me. "She writes down everything. You might end up in a book."

"Is that what you think?" I say, faking indignation. "That I only come here for material?"

She considers this. "No, you like the bagels."

My pending surgery is weighing heavily on my mind and I feel guilty about letting them think I'm only going to be off work for the next two weeks. Even though we've talked openly about everything (kids, husbands, even our sex lives), I can't bring myself to share my secret with them – not yet. Besides, they each have their own worries. Stephanie's a single mom raising teenagers alone. She had her own health scare recently, but thankfully everything is okay. Jasna has three sons, one of whom is severely developmentally delayed. At sixteen, he is non-verbal, wears diapers, and has frequent, daily seizures. Ten seizures is a good day. Janet is tackling health issues and a weight problem and has recently lost sixty pounds. "I was facing diabetes, high blood pressure, the whole kit and caboodle," she told me privately. "I took myself in hand and did something about it."

Yes, we share a lot, but today I keep quiet.

So we turn to what we always do, what we need to do, which is review the night. In order to put it all behind us, we must first go over it in detail, taking care to lower our voices and never mention patients' real names.

"I can't stay long," Stephanie warns us, as she usually does, before we begin. "I'm exhausted."

"You always say that," I remind her.

"I mean it this time. And I have to take my kids to their music lessons before I go to sleep. Tilda, you're going to have to write fast."

I start off by telling them about Simone. "She's stressed out and doesn't seem to be coping. I hope she stays — we could work with her — but she has a lot to learn."

"I hope she sees it that way," Janet says with a chuckle. "Not all of the young'uns take to our direction. Some of them act like they know it all."

Janet's words might seem harsh, if you didn't know that she's a fabulous nurse and generous mentor. And the younger nurses would likely be horrified at our critiques of their work, our strictly-in-jest, off-the-record *American Idol*–type reviews, complete with thumbs-up or -down. There's only a few we'd like to "send off the show," but even with those, we vow to help them improve their performance. We take turns being the various judges, like the dismissive critic; "That was a horrendous! Give it up, you have no talent" or more the gentle adviser: "You're not ready, dude." We lavish praise on the deserving ones: "I gotta give you major props, dog, cuz you know who you are. You're ready for the big time." We encourage those who show promise: "I see you're trying, sweetie, but you have a lot of work to do. Learn to sing first." But we revel in coming across the real deal where we can say, "That was a fabulous performance. You're going to Hollywood!"

Despite our behind-the-scenes grandstanding, we actually take a great deal of pride in nurturing new nurses and watching them blossom under our guidance. Nurses have a reputation for being hard on our young, and though they may feel like we're picking on them, we do it because we know how important it is to get everything right.

Janet is itching to tell us about her night. "It was quiet until about three, then my beeper went off. A nurse from the general surgery floor called, not sounding too concerned, but a little birdie told me I'd better go up there and have a look-see. Well, it turned out to be a good call. A middle-aged lady two days post-op bowel surgery was decompensating but fast. She was on 80 per cent O_2 but her sats were meh — so-so. I wasn't happy. She was having difficulty breathing and her pressure was in her boots, heart rate, 150. 'We already gave her a litre of fluid,' the floor nurse told me. 'Yeah, but it's not doing anything,' I said. 'You have to see if what you tried had any effect.'

"How long had her pressure been low?" Jasna asks, concern in her voice.

Low blood pressure is a huge miss.

"According to the chart, four o'clock yesterday afternoon, but no one did anything about it, only now they call me," Janet grumbles as if annoyed, but I know she's pleased she could help, maybe even save the day. "'Why didn't you call us sooner?' I ask her. 'We thought it would get better on its own,' she says. Meanwhile, the patient was confused, with a decreased level of consciousness . . ." Janet's voice trails off so that we can think through the situation ourselves and imagine what each of us would do. All the while, her fingers continue to fly, the needles clicking and clacking over the soft yarn. "I was thinking maybe she'd gotten too much sedation," Janet continues the story. "I was wondering if she needed an *anti-dope,* like Narcan."

I'm about to correct her, then realize it's a Janet-ism. Classic.

"So anyway, she's tanking and I'm thinking we'll have to tube her and bring her to the ICU. Her Ph was 7.1 . . ." She says all of this without pausing or even glancing at the lengthening swath of the intricate patterned blanket growing in her hands by the minute.

"Not good," we murmur. *Too low.* Inadequate ventilation, poor gas exchange.

"Her CO_2 was ninety and her bicarb only twelve!"

We all recognize that it's an uncompensated acid-base imbalance indicating metabolic acidosis, pending respiratory failure, and we shake our heads at the seriousness of the situation.

"She needed to be in the ICU," Jasna says in alarm, "like yesterday."

"I spoke with the ICU resident and told her that in my humble opinion . . ."

"Yeah, right," says Stephanie with a grin to Jasna and me.

". . . not only that but based on the lab work, she was dry. She needed fluids and the resident agreed, so I banged in an eighteen-gauge needle, shot in a litre and a half of saline, and you know what? She perked up in a few minutes and she might not need to be tubed after all . . ."

As they continue to discuss this complicated situation, all I can think of is that now, hearing our clipped nurse short forms anew, I realize how flippant and cavalier they must sound to outsiders. We toss these phrases off like they mean nothing, knowing they mean everything. How alienating this bravado of ours is to others, yet how necessary to us. What will it feel like to hear talk like this when I'm on the "other side of the bedrails"?

Janet looks at me. "You getting all this down, Tilda?"

"I'm quite sure she is," Stephanie says dryly. "Go on."

"So anyway, her improvement didn't last long. She quickly became completely *kaplooped,* so I arranged for her to be transferred to the ICU, but we had to get that tube in first. The respiratory therapist and ICU resident – we were all in agreement with that. The family had come in, very upset. High-strung people. Understandable. I get that. I told them I was calling a Code Blue because she needed to be tubed – stat. 'No, no, don't do that,' they said, looking terrified. To them, it meant the worst thing, but the family was watching me and they could see knew I knew what I was doing and that I was going out on a limb for their mother. They trusted me. So, we got her tubed and sedated and she looked more comfy. My work was done, but just before I left the hospital I went to the ICU for a peek. You know what? She looked better. She was in florid sepsis, but we got to her in time and she might make it."

"Good save," we congratulate her, but she doesn't easily accept the accolade.

"It's not about me – we're a team. I love being on the RRT because I need to know that patients will get what they need in their time of need."

"You sound awfully needy." Stephanie gets in one last jibe.

And this is what I will need – fearless nurses like these.

People always say they want kind, sweet, gentle nurses. That's nice, but even better are *smart* nurses who know what they're doing. If you want to survive a hospital stay, you'll need to have bold, take-charge, go-to, problem-solving nurses like these. More than *caring* nurses, you want nurses who *care,* as in *give a damn.* You need nurses who have the guts to take initiative, speak out, stand up to bullies, rattle the cage, smash hierarchies, kick up a fuss, rock the boat, and blow whistles if necessary.

But even cowboys and crusaders get tired.

Janet yawns. "I'm losing it. I'm going home to my boys." Tess, Darcy, and Mr. Bennett are her three West Highland terriers. "If I give them cookies, they'll sleep with me in bed."

"Is that how I can get a man?" Stephanie asks, stowing away her knitting.

Then it catches us all simultaneously – a wave of pure exhaustion.

"The neurons aren't firing." Jasna sticks her needles into a ball of yarn.

"Yup, the synapses have shut down," Stephanie says. "But first, Tilda will read the minutes of this meeting."

As if.

"Are we adjourned?" I ask.

"I'd say," she says and we all get up to go.

"Okay, ladies. That's it. Get to bed!" Janet calls out.

The Grand Pooh-Bah has spoken.

Toddling off to our cars, we compare HOP – Head On Pillow – time. Stephanie has to drive to music lessons so it will be a while before she sees her bed, but Jasna and Janet estimate twenty minutes, including hot showers first. Me, I can't sleep. My mind is buzzing with thoughts of warm bagels, night shifts, and good friends, wondering how many more will be allotted to me.

"Good night," we call out to one another in the bright morning light.

4

BREATHING LESSONS

On Monday, Dr. Drobac calls to tell me he's ordered a Doppler scan, similar to an ultrasound, of my neck arteries to check for atherosclerosis, which is plaque buildup in the arteries, and an angiogram to rule out coronary artery disease. All necessary preoperative tests, but *no can do.*

"I'm going away for two weeks to work at my kids' sleepover camp."

"You're symptomatic now and could get into trouble."

He means crash and burn. Sudden cardiac death.

"I'll do the tests when I get back in two weeks."

"You have to take it easy. You need surgery as soon as possible."

Unless I drop dead first. In which case I won't have to do anything.

"Have fun. Try to relax and enjoy yourself," Ivan said as I got into my car for the two-hour drive due north to the Muskoka region of Ontario. *Fat chance.* Easy for him to say. He's getting a break from me and the kids, along with extra late-night poker games and long afternoons of golf with the guys, so who's going to be enjoying themselves?

Ivan is loving – in a gruff, irascible way. He practises his own brand of "tough love" and can be hard on me. The worst was the night of the car crash when Princess Diana was killed. At around 2:00 a.m. the news broke and I was glued to the TV, in shock as I watched the aftermath of the horrific accident in a Paris tunnel. I ran to wake Ivan up and tell him.

"Princess Diana died!" I sobbed. "She's dead!"

Ivan sat up in bed and pointed his finger at me. "And you killed her! It's because of all those magazines you buy. You're as bad as the paparazzi."

You get the picture. This is what I'm dealing with.

Ivan may get emotional but never sentimental. He's not one to molly-coddle, cajole, or offer unnecessary hugs – only necessary ones. He has little tolerance for self-absorption, no patience for self-pity. He's never meditated on a mountaintop, attended an ashram, sat at the foot of a guru, nor contemplated his navel, but Ivan has attained enlightenment, albeit in his inimitable, idiosyncratic way.

In the 1980s, when I first met him, Ivan was making the seemingly trite and ubiquitous pronouncement that everyone says: "It is what it is." The thing is, Ivan really means it. He accepts whatever life brings. To Ivan, "do your best" and "don't sweat the small stuff" aren't empty platitudes; he actually lives this way. His priorities are clear: for example, when his insured clients tell him they've been in a car accident—whether it's a minor fender bender or they've totalled their car – the first question he asks and the only one he claims that matters is, "Are you okay?" Satisfied with himself, he figures if others aren't, it's their problem. He doesn't mean to offend, yet often does. In Ivan, there is a total absence of guile, malice, or spite. Though he's far from perfect – he'd be the first to admit – he accepts himself as he is. He's completely at ease with himself.

We're a good balance: he's a man of few words and I am a woman of many.

"Yes," he said twenty years ago when I asked him to marry me.

"Do you love me?" I asked.

"Of course." And that was that. What more needed to be said?

On the other hand, I do all the things he doesn't: ruminate, wonder, dream, imagine, speculate, brood, and ponder. We're so different, but somehow it works.

One evening, a few days after seeing Dr. Drobac, Ivan gives me a pep talk.

"You're going off the deep end. Get a grip. You're losing it."

"No, I'm not, but feel I might at any moment."

"Why do you always have to think the worst?"

You don't know what I've seen, I am about to say, but Ivan would see this as an excuse so I keep my mouth shut.

"You're so negative," he continues.

Yes, but only toward myself. I would never be like this with my patients. Why this double standard? I don't know.

"I hate to think how you'd react if you had something really serious."

Normally, this comment would infuriate me. It would incite me to make an angry retort, then retreat and sulk, but I'm too pre-occupied with being upset about so many other things that I can't bother to react.

"You're getting worked up for nothing," he says while taking up his post on the couch in front of the TV. TSN's *SportsCentre.* "Everything will be all right. Well get through this. Together."

I go over to sit beside him on the couch for a few minutes and stare into the TV. *If you can't beat 'em, join 'em.*

"I'm losing control of my mind," is all I can say.

"Let go and you'll actually have more control." There's a pause, since my TV Buddha dispenses his koan-bytes during commercials. "Life's tough. Deal with it."

I have to admit, these banal, maddening phrases do contain bracing truths.

At camp, doling out meds, soothing mosquito bites, removing splinters, and consoling homesick children by day – and occasionally at night – helps to keep my mind off my own problems. Most evenings, I steal away for a few minutes from my nurse partner and friend, Alice, and all the clamouring campers in the infirmary to call Vanessa.

A few days before camp started, Steven, Vanessa's husband, had a cardiac arrest and was without vital signs for almost thirty minutes. Since then he has not shown any signs of awakening. The CT scan of his head showed damage due to prolonged anoxia, or lack of oxygen, to the brain. Vanessa knows the prognosis is grim, but Steven's parents remain optimistic that he will fully recover. She spends the days at his bedside, looking for signs of life, for signs of Steven.

As soon as I arrived at camp, I realized that I had to tell Alice my secret. She needed to know why I wouldn't be running up the hill to campers' cabins or joining her for hikes in the woods or swims in the lake, as we usually do every summer. But it turns out she had noticed something was wrong with me ever since her son's bar mitzvah celebration a few months ago.

"You got up to dance and then sat right back down," Alice said. "That's so not like you, Tilda. You looked exhausted. I've been worried about you."

There's a big hill leading up to the cabins in the forest and smaller ones all over. Alice said she would do most of the legwork while I stayed put in the infirmary. Our days start early in the morning and usually finish after midnight, which is when the counsellors drop by the infirmary to chat about their own problems, restock their first-aid kits, and "chillax."

Later, that first day, when we ran through the mock emergency drill including use of the AED, the automated external defibrillator, she gave me a worried glance. She knew who's the most likely candidate at camp to need it.

Camp is fun and the kids' high-spirits cheer me up, but at night when I close the door to my cabin and lie down on my narrow cot, I return to obsessing about my heart. The wind in the pine trees outside my door, the fresh air, and beautiful lake, a few steps from the infirmary — all things that usually delight me — I barely notice. Alone with my thoughts about what lies ahead, I'm scared out of my mind.

Anxiety rises up in waves of panic. Often I get up and work on "The List," a growing inventory of fears. I fill one notebook, then another, no matter how outlandish or far-fetched, with everything I'm afraid of about this experience ahead of me. After one week at camp I have quite the list. I read through it, feeling a shiver of fear with each item.

- *Not being here for my kids!* Harry at the flagpole this evening kept his distance from me — wouldn't even say hi. Thirteen years old, he's acting like a typical teenager, but it hurts. Maybe it won't be so bad for them if I'm not around. What if I make it but am unable to take care of them? What good is that? A lung transplant patient told me how hard she worked to hide her infirmity from her son. "I never wanted him to see me, you know, on oxygen."

"Did he?"

"Yes," she admitted, "but that's all he saw, me on oxygen."
Harry is on to me. For some time, he's noticed that something
is wrong with me. For Mother's Day he made me a card by
photo-shopping my head on to Lance Armstrong's body out in
front of the pack in the Tour de France, with a gently sarcastic
caption about my athletic prowess. Harry knows way more
than he lets on. Max at eleven years knows what he knows
and lets you know it. He came by today to say hey and make
me laugh. "It's my job, Mom." Harry's quiet jokes creep up on
me unawares while Max's are out in the open. They'll be fine
without me. They'll survive. Besides, they're always complaining
about my food. Mom burnt the soup again, etc. Ivan is a
much better cook.

- Cardiac catheterization! Invasive and uncomfortable, but
  worse than the procedure is the results. If I have blocked arteries,
  I will need a bypass as well as a valve replacement.
- A screw-up! Too many possibilities to enumerate.
- Complications My own body letting me down! Ditto.
- Surgeon Having an Off Day — I went to a hairdresser
  once who said that sometimes he just didn't feel like it —
  cutting hair, that is. What if your surgeon isn't in the mood
  that day?
- Cracking open my ribcage! Sternum cut, ribcage pulled
  apart, chest cavity cracked open. The deepest invasion.
- Going under! Where will I be? Gone! The void! A black hole.
  The lost time! An anesthesiologist friend I know once told me
  that every patient asks if they will wake up. "It's my job to
  make sure of that," he says.

   Another friend told me that a radio was playing in the
operating room as she was being wheeled in for surgery. The

> moment before she went under, her last memory before the
> lights went out was the opening bars of "Stairway to Heaven."
>
> • The visuals! The splash of red, the blue OR scrubs, the steel
>   instruments probing inside my body. This is what is meant by
>   the expression "going under the knife."
> • The soundtrack! Hushed voices surround the grey, anesthetized
>   body (me!) on the operating table, the whoosh of the ventilator
>   breathing for me, the sucking of spilled blood to salvage my own
>   red cells so, I hope, I won't need a blood transfusion.

My mind has gone wild, but keeping things in perspective has
never been my strong suit. I close my notebook and think about a
friend of mine, Daphne, who died of cancer. All the time she was
ill, she never allowed herself a single negative thought. "I don't
permit them in," she would say, laughing at her diagnosis. She
refused to believe she was dying; even at the moment of her death,
she remained unconvinced. Her optimism was admirable, for sure,
but it's not me – at least not yet. First, I have to face this head-on,
eyes open, knowing all the details, and then still choose to go forward with it. Being naively positive feels like I'm deluding myself.

I call Vanessa again the following week. It's now been three weeks
since Steven's cardiac arrest and he remains deeply comatose.
Vanessa doesn't know whether to hope for improvement or to
begin to let go. "What would Steven want?" she asks herself. It's
the right question to ask; its answer will guide her to advocate in a
way that is in keeping with Steven's values and beliefs. The doctors
have explained that he'd been without oxygen for so long that his
brain is permanently damaged. He's off the ventilator now, just on
an oxygen mask, so he's been transferred from the ICU to a step-
down unit.

My thoughts are with Steven, but I can't help but think of my situation, too. For years, I've talked about scenarios like these with Ivan, always in connection with patients. I'm not certain he knows my end-of-life wishes, nor do I about him. Do most spouses? Here's yet another thing to add to my growing "to do" list: have that difficult conversation with Ivan. Just in case.

This summer, I'm preoccupied with my own problem and can't muster my usual patience with campers, especially Kevin, an intense and inquisitive eleven-year-old who comes every morning for ADD meds and badgers me with queries and observations.

"I have a question," he starts off, thinking out loud and gazing around at all the packages and bottles of other campers' meds. "What's that one for?" "How many pills do you have here? "Where do you sleep?" "Do you give needles?" I'm relieved when his counsellor leads him away to breakfast. "I have a question," I hear him saying as he walks past the window toward the dining hall. "Do you think the nurse will let me try out her stethoscope? Can I ask her later?"

I admit it. I have a soft spot for the kids with headaches, the anxious and the homesick, probably because I've had these conditions myself. It's harder for me to be sympathetic about splinters, warts, and bumps, bruises, or little cuts, since those things don't bother me and I don't pay much attention to them even when they affect my own children. So often empathy comes out of your personal experience, but it shouldn't be that way, especially not for nurses who are *professional empathizers*. "Empathy" makes us good at what we do and is one of the main tools of our trade. We expect ourselves to be able to conjure it up and provide it for all who are in our care — we are equal-opportunity empathizers — or at least we are supposed to be, but it's not an easy gig. One nurse I know always seems to lavish extra care and attention on HIV-positive patients ever since her own brother was diagnosed with same thing. A new graduate becomes an oncology nurse in the aftermath of her mother's death from lung cancer; she has a need to experience or explore something personal through her work. We're not supposed to have such biases or allow our own issues to affect our nursing care, but the reality is that sometimes we do.

Empathy can be a challenge at times, even at camp. Sometimes I wonder at the different responses of children. There are some kids who get upset about relatively minor things such as a bug bite while others seem unconcerned about a fever or even a fracture. Parents' reactions can be just as idiosyncratic and unpredictable, like the mother I called about her son's infected rash that the doctor wanted to treat with an antibiotic. She seemed surprised that we'd bother to call her at all about something she considered trivial. For my part, I was surprised at her calm response, but it made sense when she happened to mention she was a nurse – a cardiovascular anesthesiologist first assistant.

"Can you do everything an anesthesiologist does?" I inquire.

"Yes, except get paid like one," she says ruefully.

I hesitate but have to ask. "Have you ever assisted in the OR with valve replacements?"

"Yes, many."

"How do these patients do, generally speaking?" I say casually, covertly trawling for insider information.

"Most do very well. Why do you ask?"

"Just wondering."

It is the middle of the night and I bolt up out of bed, my heart pounding, my mind racing. I pull out my notebook, intent on recording each fear, the rational and legit ones, all mixed together with the bizarre and nonsensical. I explore each one in order to weaken its hold over me, in the hope that this list will eventually come to an end.

- *Cardioplegia* – *Stopping my Heart. It's done with a lethal injection of potassium chloride, but how do they start it up again? What if it wants to keep on resting? The cardiac monitor will show a flatline. That's not a mere blip on the screen! What a world of difference there is between*

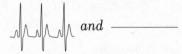 *and* ───────

  It's not merely "life" versus "death," it's alive versus dead. A walking, talking person versus a cold and still body.
- *The Heart-Lung Bypass Machine. Too much or too little blood thinner, air bubble in the tubing causing an embolism, or a machine malfunction. My life will be dependent on a machine, even more on the perfusionist, the person operating it.*
- *Being awake during the surgery. The horror of being locked in, aware of them cutting into me, and not being able to let them know. It's a rare but not-unheard-of phenomenon.*
- *Not waking up afterward. If I die, I won't even know I've died. Everyone will know but me. I will be left out of the loop. It seems unfair.*
- *That I will wake up but . . . That I'll be in an impaired state, cognitively damaged or weirdly different, a burden to my family, a "cardiac cripple."*
- *Loss of dignity. I will lose control of myself. Families always say their loved one is never like that. "Dad is so gentle. He would never hurt anyone," a daughter said in shock after watching her father kick at a nurse, yell obscenities, and try to climb out of bed.*

- *The surrender. It's a total loss of control. I'll be at the mercy of others taking care of me. All I will have to go on is faith and fate.*
- *The allure of despair – What if I don't fight to survive? What if my survival instinct isn't sufficiently tenacious? If I was adrift at sea or trapped in a burning building, how hard would I fight to save my life? I've never been confident of my answer.*
- *Death – Part II – In our household, the word "bored" is forbidden, but I have to admit, death does sound boring. I'll be missing out on everything!*
- *The irretrievable loss of time. Something important is being done to my most vital organ and I'm going to be sleeping through it, unavailable for the main event and will have no memory of it. "À la recherché du temps perdue," as Marcel Proust said.*

I look over my list. It covers most eventualities, but I am compelled to continue because according to the rules of my magical thinking, I must exhaust every possibility of disaster in order to avoid it.

This is a very progressive camp. It has a psychologist on staff by the name of Dr. John Fleming who gives sessions on stress management and relaxation techniques to anxious, over-scheduled campers and their equally stressed counsellors. He teaches them something called mindfulness meditation. After one week of sleepless nights, I cornered him after lunch today to ask for a private lesson. He agreed to meet with me at the picnic table under a big tree near the dining hall later this afternoon. Mindfulness? Sounds interesting, but can it help me in my situation? I am ready to hear what he has to say, but I'm a New Age skeptic.

The moment I sit down opposite John at the picnic table, I fall apart. Something about him makes me feel completely safe and I don't hold back. Up until now, I haven't cried, but in front of him, I allow myself to weep and wail and say all the dire, drastic things I've only been thinking and scribbling in my notebooks. He listens closely and intensely in a way I've never experienced. His listening is breaking me wide open.

He shows no reaction to what I'm saying. There's no expression of concern or worry so I don't have to protect or console him as I would a friend, yet he is not detached nor disinterested. Around my age, he's also a parent of young children but doesn't interject with his own feelings or identify in anyway with my problem. He doesn't appear to be making a diagnosis, or judging me or drawing any conclusions. He offers no advice or suggestions. He sits implacably, radiating a benevolent kindness, an unwavering interest in my situation and respect for what I'm going through.

I finish crying and am ready to hear what he has to say.

"The basic principle of mindfulness is that rather than expend effort to fend off our pain, we simply stay aware of what we are feeling and thinking. Each time your mind goes to a fear, breathe and bring your attention to your breath."

Is that it? Is this all you've got?

He goes on to explain that mindfulness keeps the heart soft and accepting. It is a way to focus the mind on the present so that you can be fully awake and aware to what is happening in this moment, now, without judgment. It cultivates a gentle friendliness to what is. It's not a religion or a doctrine, but a practice of conscious breathing and meditation.

"Let's begin," he says. "Take off your sandals. Let your feet feel the ground."

I do as he says and await further instructions.

"Don't run from your feelings. Breathe into them. Feel whatever comes up, panic, fear, sadness, whatever. Sit and observe each thought as it comes and as it goes. See how you can survive each feeling and watch how it passes on its own."

I try it for a few minutes but lose patience.

"Perhaps there's a book you could recommend about meditation?" *One day I'll meditate, I promise, but not now! I don't have time for this.*

Note to self: Google mindfulness, meditation, serenity, etc.

We're meeting again tomorrow. It's a lot of work, this breathing.

It's Day Two in Mindfulness lessons with John and I bring my lists to show him what we're dealing with here, including last night's entry:

- *Intubation. That tube down my throat, in my lungs, breathing for me, the sensation of choking. Many patients say it's the worst part. What if I pull out the tube by accident as some agitated patients do and wreck my vocal cords?*
- *Dying on the table. The surgeon comes out, slowly makes his way over to Ivan and the kids, and solemnly says, "We did everything we could . . . I'm sorry . . . but she's gone." Boo-hoo.*
- *Death Part III – Death is bad, but dying can be worse.*
- *The scar. An ugly, permanent souvenir running down the length of my chest.*
- *Loss of privacy. When pesky Kevin asked me questions about another camper's meds I explained about privacy and the "circle of care," meaning that only the people caring for that child have the right to know this information. I love my privacy, too, but it's likely I'll be a patient in the hospital where I've worked as a nurse for twenty-five years! I know everyone*

and everyone knows me. My secret insides will be exposed.
Others will see parts of my body that I'll never get to see.
They'll see me naked! They'll see my urine – even worse –
they'll know my weight!

John gives my notebook a glance and sets it aside on the picnic table, which makes me realize that the particulars of my situation are not what this exercise is about; it's about fear itself. We return to the work of breathing. I take a desperate gulp of air like it's my last.

"Let it out, too," John reminds me. "With each feeling that arises, surrender to it. Identify each fear, then let it go. Meet it with compassion for yourself."

My mind is full of scary thoughts. "Bad stuff keeps coming up."

"Escort each unwelcome guest to the door. Note the thought and the feelings it creates, then let them go."

I sit with that for a minute or two. My eyes pop open. "Just to recap, what's the *purpose* of all of this?"

"To bring us back to the present, to an awareness of this moment, which is all we have."

I look up at the sunlight shining down through the trees making them so bright and green. The blue lake peeks through the leafy branches, sparkling in the breeze. I understand that what I'm looking at is beautiful, but I can't connect with it – I barely see it. It's as if I'm not even here. I'm already on the operating table, the surgeon's scalpel poised above my chest, about to cut into me.

"Should I keep my eyes open? Closed? Assume the lotus position?"

"It doesn't matter. Just sit and be aware of what is right here now."

"Hey, John. I'm sorry. I can't do this. I don't want to waste any more of your time. Meditation is not for me."

"Just breathe," he encourages me, "in and out."

I can't still my chattering mind. I strain to hear him over the static in my head.

"What are you feeling?"

"Terrified!"

"Pay attention to how your thoughts create your feelings."

I close my eyes. "Am I meditating yet?" I ask after a few more minutes.

"We're not there yet. It may take a lifetime to master."

Who has time for this?

I open my eyes. "This isn't working." He doesn't get it. He's not the one who has to go under the knife, have his chest cracked open, his heart stopped. I look at his kind face, his fit, athletic body. Every morning, he goes for a ride in the countryside on his mountain bike. What does he know about physical limitations? I shake my head. "I have to get back to work. Keeping busy is the only thing that helps me."

The next morning I am practising my own brand of meditation as I treat the kids' various ailments. I put a bandage on a kid's arm and breathe in deeply. I give an antihistamine for a case of hives. A wave of panic washes over me and I wait and watch it subside. The kids push to the front of the line, each wanting to be seen first. I treat them and momentarily they're satisfied. But there is one child whose need is endless.

"I have a question," Kevin starts up again. I try to ignore him.

"Can I try your stethoscope?" he asks.

"No," I snap at him, all serenity vanished.

"Why do the pills come in different colours? What do they taste like? Are there flavours? What's the strongest one?"

"In the wrong dose, they all can kill you." I shoot him a menacing glare. *Scram, kid.*

"I have a question."

"Just one?"

"Yes."

"What is it?"

"Can I ask you privately?"

"Of course."

"Do I have to make an appointment?"

"No. How about right now?" *I have a question, too. Does this kid do anything but ask questions?*

We go outside and sit on the grass and I wait for the question.

"I don't know what's wrong with me, but I'm not having a good time at camp. What can I do to help myself feel better?"

I look at him, his freckled face focused on mine. This is a good question! Now we're getting somewhere! We talk for an hour and plan strategies. He will focus more on the activities he enjoys, cross off days on the calendar, and come for daily talks with me. I will arrange with his counsellor for him to have downtime, some quiet and privacy that there is so little of at camp. My advice is practical, but maybe John's approach could also help him to feel better. I will arrange for them to meet tomorrow. Kevin returns to his cabin in better spirits, as I do to mine.

My stint at camp is finished. My kids are staying for another week and a half, but it's time for me to go home and face the music — *Open-Heart Surgery: The Musical.*

Alice and I go to our cars and she asks as she always does at the end of our time at camp, just as we are saying goodbye, "Will you come back next year?"

"Yeah, if I'm still alive."

She laughs, assuming it's a joke. She doesn't for a minute think I'm going to die. Probably not, but there are many other possibilities.

"You're strong. You'll make it," Alice says, echoing Mary.

"We'll see about that." I hug her and try to commit her embrace to memory.

A few days after I'm home from camp, I go to the hospital to visit Steven. Outside his door stands Albie, his elderly father, who looks like he should be the patient. Stooped over and breathing heavily with chronic lung disease, he's had congestive heart failure, diabetes, and lots of aches and pains for years yet keeps on keeping on. "They're going to have to shoot me," he always says.

He brightens when he sees me. "Pssst . . ." he says, waving me over. "Here's a hot tip. D'you wanna sell more books? Put in a centrefold. I'll even pose for it. How 'bout it?"

I'm so familiar with this old-man Jewish humour that it doesn't bother me, even at a time like this. It comes from a long cultural tradition of laughing through the pain.

"How're you doing, Albie?"

"Steven is sick, but he'll be just fine, don't you worry. As for me, I've never felt better! I have a bowel movement every morning at 7:00. Problem is, I wake up at 7:30."

I can't help but laugh, but then remember something. "You had a bypass, didn't you, Albie? When was that?"

"Take a guess."

"2000?"

"Close. 1986. Quadruple. Yup, I'm a charter member of the Zipper Club." He lifts up his shirt to show me the long scar on his chest.

"What was it like?"

"A piece of cake! A walk in the park! My problem is I'm having too much sex."

"Shhh . . . !" Carol, Albie's wife, admonishes him.

Albie may be in high spirits, but Vanessa knows the score and she's worried. "Steven looks terrible," she says. "Please go in there and tell me what's happening."

As soon as I go in I understand. What's happening is that Steven is crashing. His systolic blood pressure is hovering in the seventies, with his mean arterial pressure in the fifties. (In the ICU, we usually aim for at least a MAP of sixty millimetres of mercury (mmHg), the absolute minimum necessary to provide blood flow to the coronary arteries, brain, and kidneys.) Steven is gasping, hungry for air. Even worse is that his heart has slowed down to around fifty-five beats per minute. A healthy heart responds to stress by speeding up to maintain cardiac output. The nurses sit, chatting. When they get up and move, their feet are in cement. This man has a very poor prognosis, but at this point he is a *full code.*

"Hey, listen up!" I clap my hands to get their attention. "This man is in trouble. He needs central IV access, an arterial line, fluids, intubation!"

"Are you family?" one nurse asks.

"Yes," I say, after a nod from Vanessa. "This is an impending arrest," I say, stating the obvious. From the nurses, there's no response. Why aren't they doing anything? "Where's the doctor?" I ask.

"I have no idea." Steven's nurse bends down to empty the urine bag for 1600 hours and dutifully charts the two drops she manages to squeeze out of the urometer.

Steven's kidneys are shutting down, but even more pressing is that his oxygen saturation has plummeted to 74 per cent. "Turn up his oxygen!"

The nurse says she doesn't know how and even if she did, they aren't allowed to adjust oxygen flow. Steven's blood pressure is dropping farther. He needs fluids and probably an inotrope to constrict his vessels and boost his pressure. I don't trust the blood pressure reading on the cardiac monitor because the wave form is dampened, so I go over to take his blood pressure myself the old-fashioned way, with a cuff and stethoscope that's hanging on the IV pole. It's barely detectable. But the systolic is around sixty, lower than what it shows on the monitor screen. *Steven's heart is dying before our very eyes.*

His nurse sits at a desk, busy with her charting, probably writing something like, *Difficult visitor. Will call Security to remove visitor if disruptive behaviour continues.* The other nurse pretends to be very busy, tucking the covers around an elderly patient, settling him in for a nap. How to wake them up, galvanize them into action? I don't care if I'm out of line. People die because of this kind of indifference, this antiquated view some nurses have of themselves that they are helpless or powerless.

But I rein myself in and soften my tone to be more diplomatic.

"You might want to call the doctor," I say gently.

"He's busy," the nurse answers.

"Tell him the patient is crashing. He's about to arrest."

She glares at me. From across the room, the other nurse stares at me. Their expressions seem to say, *We're just nurses. There's nothing we can do. What if the doctor gets angry at us?* They've given up. If I wasn't so caught up in the situation and my feelings for Steven, I could actually muster some sympathy for them. I was a nurse like this, once. I remember feeling so constrained and afraid. I know the frustration of seeing problems but not having the means to fix them.

And it's not all that unusual that big, obvious signs of trouble like this get wildly missed. Unfortunately, it's been known to happen and it's one of the reasons that the Rapid Response Teams were created in hospitals. There's even a name for this kind of situation: failure to rescue. Sometimes it occurs when doctors don't listen to nurses, but here, the nurses aren't even speaking up to the doctor on behalf of their patient.

"Page the Rapid Response Team!" I demand.

"We don't have one yet, we're still developing it."

Precious minutes go by, but at last the nurse tells Vanessa the doctor is coming and they've called the respiratory therapist to assist with intubation. Steven's blood pressure is still low, but he's responding to a bolus of saline that the nurse finally started. They've gotten the ball rolling. It may be too little, too late, but Steven's condition seems stable for now. It's time for me to go home.

"Is he going to make it?" Albie asks when I come out of the room.

"I think so," I say wearily, "for now, anyway."

I get home, turn on *Dr. Phil,* open a bottle of wine, and start dinner. It's romantic, having the house to ourselves, like old times.

Soon, I hear Ivan's car in the garage, then his key in the door, and I get that familiar flutter. Did I happen to mention how handsome Ivan is, in a rogue-ish, pirate-y sort of way? Short, strong, swarthy, and rough-looking, he's completely my type. *Would I be able to have sex, one last time?* I greet him as the phone rings. It's Sue, Vanessa's neighbour from across the street. She had arrived at the hospital just as I was leaving, less than an hour ago.

"Steven died. He went into cardiac arrest just after you left. They called a Code Blue and worked on him for almost an hour, but he didn't make it."

Now I know what my biggest fear is. It's the best-kept hospital secret. Nurses are capable of the greatest good and also the greatest harm. They will cure or kill me – or worse. They will protect or neglect me, save or sabotage me. The worst thing to have if you're a patient is a scared, cowardly nurse, one who sees a problem but looks away and does nothing, a timid nurse who's afraid to go out on a limb or an indifferent one who doesn't care enough and gives up.

To survive this experience, I will need nurses caring for me who have guts and grit; smart, staunch, stubborn, protective, feisty, fierce nurses, savvy nurses with moxie, pluck, and chutzpah. I'll take a brave nurse over a nice one any day! Patients always say they want the best doctor, the most qualified, the top of the class. Fair enough, but they rarely give a thought to the quality or qualifications of the nurses who will be caring for them. This is a dangerous oversight because nurses are the ones who will keep you safe – or not. They are in charge of seeing that you get better. The problem is they are the salvation and the danger, both the rescue and the risk – and possibly the weakest link.

5

TICKING TIME BOMB

Chocolate doughnuts, double-cheese pizzas, Rocky Road ice cream, and other sugary and trans-fat-laden delights – I'm on the phone confessing all my dietary transgressions to Mary and am coming to the realization that my *carbohydrate foodprint* is more damning than my carbon footprint.

"But what about the olives!" Mary reminds me, in my defence.

She's got a point. In my refrigerator right now, there's a jar of dry, wrinkled black olives from Morocco, containers of green, Spanish ones stuffed with chipotle peppers, and smooth-skinned, dark Kalamata from Greece, chock full of vitamins, omega 3s, and antioxidants. Also on my kitchen shelves are walnuts, blueberries, and bran. Does it balance out? Risk factors and lifestyle choices – each only half of the picture.

I didn't completely come clean with Dr. Drobac: I do have a significant cardiac family history. My father had coronary artery disease, which caused him frequent bouts of crushing chest pain (angina) for which he popped nitroglycerin pills like candy. He ignored his doctor's advice to lose weight, even when he eventually developed diabetes and had to go on insulin. At sixty-two, he had a massive heart attack that caused cardiac arrest and he died. My eating habits are also bad and I'm always carrying around an extra twenty (more like thirty) pounds. I guess I've been in denial about that, too, because I seem to have the opposite problem than most women, always thinking I'm thinner and fitter than I really am.

Inexplicably and undeservedly, my test results came back perfect. My blood sugar is normal, my good cholesterol is high, and the bad is low. But tomorrow is the big reveal: a cardiac angiogram is the ultimate report card. If there are blockages in my coronary arteries, that's a failing grade. It means I will need a bypass as well as a valve replacement and will require an even longer, more difficult surgery with greater risks and potential for complications.

"Tilda, if you had stayed, could you have saved Steven?" Albie asks me.

"I'm sorry. I wish I could have, but . . . no."

Steven had massive irreversible heart and brain damage. He couldn't be saved, but the nurses and doctors didn't even try. But what about patients who do need rescuing – a patient like me, for example? Will they give up on me, too? Will important things be missed? Will my nurses fight for me?

Albie is looking for answers, trying to fathom the death of his son. As hard as it if for her, Vanessa seems more accepting of the situation. She knew how sick Steven was and, given his underlying medical problems coupled with such extensive brain damage, how unlikely was the chance of any significant recovery. She knows Steven wouldn't have wanted to live under those circumstances, but what disturbs her is that he died in such a violent and undignified way. A Code Blue involves pounding on the chest, possible cracking of ribs, often electric shocks, and possibly other extreme measures but, in this case, futile efforts.

It's the day after, and according to Jewish law, the burial must take place as soon as possible. I'm helping Vanessa with funeral arrangements, the shiva, and keeping it all together.

At the cemetery, Albie gets out of the hearse slowly. When he sees me, he says sadly, "You spend your life stopping at red lights, but when you're dead they let you go right through them." Together, we follow the ancient custom of tossing a shovel-full of earth onto the casket. I put my arm around his back that sags with grief. "No matter how you work and strive, you don't get out of life alive," he says.

"You're a poet, Albie."

"And don't even know it."

One day, these corny, old jokes will be gone, too.

We stand at the graveside, each of us with a damaged heart: Albie's is failing, Vanessa's is broken, Steven's is dead, and mine, defective.

At the house with the other mourners, I stay near Vanessa, as close as she'll let me. She wants to be alone, to grieve by herself, but it's not allowed. Jews have a tradition of insisting on communal mourning.

"Many people have unhappy marriages," she tells me privately. "We didn't. Steven and I had our problems, but we loved each other. We enjoyed each other's company."

It showed.

I've done the neck vein ultrasound, more blood work, and have just undergone the most thorough examination in my life by a nurse practitioner (NP), who prodded and palpated every part of my body and reviewed my entire health history. I hadn't weighed myself in a while, so the number on the scale takes me aback, but she merely notes it without judgment. "Our focus used to be on the scale, but now it's the measuring tape," she explains, placing one around my waist. She's more concerned about my waist circumference, which is a few inches more than the thirty-five considered normal for women (or forty for men), than she is about the extra pounds I carry. My basal metabolic rate is in the "moderately overweight range" with my fat deposits around the waist and belly making me a classic "apple." It's much better to have the healthier "pear" shape. My excess abdominal adipose means I have a greater likelihood of developing diabetes, high blood pressure, and certain types of cancer. Scary to contemplate.

The NP shares an office with the cardiologist who will do the angiograms. On the wall, I happen to see a framed letter from Elvis, return address "Graceland." Interesting. I always like to know something personal about the people caring for me.

Afterward, back at home, I call Mary to report to her the results of the neck vein test. "My carotid arteries are clear." Less risk of stroke. One bit of good news. I should be more cheerful, but I'm still glum.

"Lucky they didn't check your head. That'd be clear as mud," she says in her Maritime twang.

It's the night before the angiogram and I practise sitting calmly and breathing through my anxiety. *Don't try to get rid of fear or escape from bad feelings,* John had said. *Sit still. Lean into them. Note each thought as it arises and then let it go. When feelings arise, observe them. Pay attention to your breathing. Ride each breath.* I use these techniques to try to tame my wild mind, but an endless stream of bad thoughts, like wedding crashers, keep intruding. Yet, during the few fleeting moments when I do stay in the present and focus on my breaths, I'm not flooded with terror. How to sustain this Zen-like state? It takes practice, John kept reminding me.

Yes, learning to be mindful does takes intention and effort. It is much easier and more familiar to default to anxiety and worry. Now I have a better understanding of women who choose to go through childbirth without painkillers. "Go toward the pain," birth coaches and midwives advise. The idea is that the pain will bring about the baby's delivery and ultimately the mother's relief, too. You have to be brave to want that pain, even ask for it. For my births, I didn't go *au naturel,* but for this experience, I feel a need to stay wide awake and face it head-on, not numb my feelings.

But I keep thinking of Charlotte, an old friend from the ICU who I ran into recently at the hospital. She'd just gotten engaged. I didn't even know she was dating anyone, but it was like her to be ultra secret about her private life. I'd been working beside her in the ICU the day we heard over the loudspeaker: "Code Blue. Cardiac Angiogram Suite." Her body jolted and her hands trembled as she tried to compose herself. "My mother is having an angiogram." She looked at her watch. "Right about now. I was going to see her after it was over."

"Go now. I'll cover your patient for you."

"Mom's okay, Mom's okay," I heard her whisper to herself.

By the time she got there, a full resuscitation was underway. Her mother arrested during the angiogram. When Charlotte arrived, they had just pronounced her dead.

Two months later, Charlotte returned to work but clearly wasn't ready because at the end of the day she resigned. She now works in Nursing Information Systems.

After a restless sleep, the next morning I arrive early at the hospital for my angiogram. I have banished Ivan from coming with me because he's terrible at waiting. He paces around, drinks too much coffee, makes phone calls, and keeps checking the clock. I told him to go to the office and I'll call him to pick me up when it's done. He gave me a quick hug – this, a necessary one – and rushed off, relieved to be off-duty. It's good. I want to keep my family out of the hospital. No one should spend time here unless they have to.

I'm assigned to a stretcher in a bay and sit on it in my flimsy gown and wait. Waiting is always involved. I expect to wait. I can't add waiting to my stress, on top of everything else. They tell you ten minutes? Count on an hour. You have to be patient to be a patient. Waiting is time to practise my new hobby, mindfulness. I breathe and slow down my mind, which if left unchecked, races in circles.

It's not working! This stuff is for the birds.

A small group of student nurses approaches me, holding out their copies of *A Nurse's Story* for me to sign. They'd seen my name on the patient roster. "Is it you?" they ask, even though I have the kind of name that's unlikely to be mistaken for anyone else's. It's a nice diversion and of course so flattering to be recognized that I overlook this minor breach of confidentiality.

Waiting with other patients for our angiograms, we lie on gurneys, lined up like cars in a parking lot. I strike up a conversation with my neighbour and his glamorous wife, Esmé. At sixty-five, Edward is a sailor and golfer. He has no symptoms and was taken by surprise when his doctor told him at a yearly checkup that he had valve disease. His was caused by ordinary wear and tear, not faulty from birth, like mine. He's an engineer who works in "predictive maintenance," estimating the lifespan of industrial machinery, calculating depreciation, and deciding on repair or replacement. I can't help but draw a comparison to the situation he and I find ourselves in with our own internal mechanisms.

I've never worked in this part of the hospital and don't know any of these nurses, nor them me, which is just as well. A nurse comes over and introduces herself to me as Nurse Louellen. She takes my vital signs, looking preoccupied and distracted. I ask her what's wrong and she tells me that she is worried about her back. She has a doctor's appointment today after work. Nurse Zahra is taking care of Edward and I hear her outlining exactly what the angiogram will involve, explaining that a catheter will be inserted into the femoral artery in his groin and dye will be injected. I listen in to the conversation because even though I know this information, it's soothing to hear it explained in simple terms.

When Dr. Sternberg comes to meet me, we chat first about Elvis, "Jailhouse Rock," and "Heartbreak Hotel," from which he segues straight into the risks of angiograms: heart attack, arrhythmias, bleeding, clots, infection, adverse reactions to sedation or to the dye, and cardiac arrest. With a bouncing, eager energy and a boyish grin, he's positively jovial. This is a man who loves his work. I consent to it all and sign on the dotted line. *Bring it on.*

"Is this your first time performing this procedure?" I tease him.

"On you it is," he says with a wink.

He's eager to get started. There are about ten of us. Now we're more like idling cars awaiting test drives, our motors revving.

"Do you have any questions?" he asks before rushing off.

"No. No questions, I just want to tell you something." He stops to listen. "If something bad happens . . . If there's no chance of survival . . . I don't want my life sustained on machines."

"No one does," he says, leaving me to muse on his true, but cryptic, answer.

When they wheel me into the angiogram suite, it's so cold that I imagine I can see my frosted breath. If I didn't know they kept these rooms like a freezer and the reasons – to prevent growth of bacteria and to minimize bleeding – the sudden chill would be shock. A technician places a heavy lead blanket over me for protection from the radiation.

"I'm going to give you some light sedation," Dr. Sternberg says.

"I'd rather not have it," I tell him. *I can't lose control.*

"I'd recommend it. I'd have sedation if it were me undergoing this procedure," he says cheerfully while a nurse cleans the area and places sterile drapes over the lower half of my body. I agree to a local anesthetic only and in the opening of the drapes, he finds the right spot and freezes the area. Yes, for a few moments there is an intense pain, but I take it like the spiritual warrior I am aspiring to be. *Push through the pain,* John said. *Breathe.*

At first, Dr. Sternberg has difficulty locating my artery, probably because my pulse is weak.

"Oh, I'll find it," he says confidently. "I've had bigger challenges than this."

Soon, I feel the needle deep inside me, where arteries lie, not superficial, like veins. Then, suddenly, on the fluoroscopy screen on the wall to the left of me, I come face to face with my own heart.

Oh, hello there. What a wondrous sight. Tucked away, undercover, out of sight, you've been working hard all these years. Taking care of business. Finally, we get to meet. Steady there, old dog. Don't stop now. Please keep it up.

Dr. Sternberg keeps up a running patter of commentary for my entertainment and edification. As he injects the dye, he points out the main arteries – the right coronary, the circumflex, and the left anterior descending (also known by its ominous nickname, "the widow-maker," because if that artery gets suddenly blocked, by atherosclerotic plaque for example, for which middle-aged men are at a higher risk, it causes a massive heart attack and usually sudden death). But he has left out the most important information – what really matters – can he see any blockages?

"Now I'm going to inject dye into the aortic root to measure your valve. It may cause an *unusual* sensation," he warns me with a sly grin.

Wow. Suddenly, I am flooded with warmth . . . down there. It feels like . . . a hot flash, but *down there.*

He grins behind his mask with a twinkle in his eyes. "I had a patient once, an elderly lady, who said when I did that, 'I think I'm having an *organism.*'"

When it's done, he gives me a partial verdict. "Your valve is point-seven square centimetres. That's a severe constriction and explains your symptoms. Surgery is indicated for anything less than one square centimetre."

"Could I suddenly arrest? Am I a walking time bomb?" *Kaboom!*

"We all are," he says quite cheerfully as he peels off his gloves and disposes of them. It sounds blunt, but again, it's honest and I appreciate his directness and unexpected humour. He gives a huge grin and hustles off to the next case.

They wheel me back to my stall and place a C-clamp on my groin with firm pressure to stop the bleeding from the artery. Nurse Louellen checks my pulses and compares my legs. "The doctor will come and tell you the rest of the results," she says and goes on her coffee break. A few minutes later, Nurse Zahra, who's covering for Louellen, comes in to assess and palpate my pulses. She looks closely at my feet and legs and notes some mottling in the right one so she loosens the clamp to ease up the pressure, all the while explaining what she is doing. Why can't I have Nurse Zahra instead of Nurse Louellen? Both are competent, but Nurse Zahra is fabulous. One inspires confidence and the other not so much; one communicates well, the other, not. I never realized just how closely patients watch nurses' every move, hang on to every word. Maybe I once knew, but over the years, it's easy to forget.

Dr. Sternberg moves down the row of patients, giving his reports. Some patients need to have angioplasty to open up narrowed arteries and others are getting stents, an artificial device used to keep the arteries open.

"Partially blocked," he tells an elderly man in the bed beside me, "but no surgery at this time. We'll keep an eye on it. Diet, exercise . . . same as last year."

Then it's my turn. Dr. Sternberg appears at the foot of my stretcher with my results. "Your arteries are perfectly clear. No blockages."

I sink down in a huge exhalation, peacefully jubilant, quietly ecstatic, containing my happiness. "Thank you," I say, as if he's responsible for the results as well as the procedure. I clasp his hand. "Thank you," I repeat. "Thank God," I say softly, putting it out there, testing it out.

"You're welcome." He says goodbye, leaving me to muse over which of my thank yous he was accepting.

Yes, if I knew how to go about it, I would offer up a prayer of gratitude. You can't go through something like this and not *occasionally* think about God because if you want to give thanks, who are you thanking? Personally, I don't allow myself to pray for specific outcomes, but I do feel moved to say "thanks" from time to time. Until now, gratitude felt impossible, but now it's here. I've spent these past three weeks being worried and now this is hope. No wonder everyone wants a piece of it.

I am beginning to think I actually might make it, but still, I take nothing for granted.

Nurse Louellen brings me a cheese sandwich. Peeling off the plastic wrapper, I'm suddenly ravenous. I take a bite into what is quite possibly the most delicious thing I've ever tasted. I feel myself turning a corner. I'm feeling great, relishing my state of quiet rapture until a new worry occurs to me – one I hadn't even thought about. How long will I have to wait for surgery? I've heard stories of long wait times for urgent procedures, even surgeries, and like every patient, *I want it now.*

I ask Nurse Louellen about this and in answer she hands me a brochure about a cardiac surgery hotline I can call if I have any concerns. "The cardiac care network ensures that all cardiac patients receive the best and most timely care," it states in the brochure. Even though wait times for cardiac procedures have improved over the past few years, it's easy to fall through the cracks and get missed, but like a good citizen, I'm determined to play by the rules. I don't want special treatment and refuse to pull in my connections. I'll let it play out as it will. I am counting on being able to trust that I'll get what I need when I need it.

In preparation for me to go home, Nurse Louellen lists the warning signs for complications post-angiogram over the next twenty-four hours but stops with a laugh. "Why am I telling you? You're an ICU nurse? You know all of this, don't you?"

"Tell me anyway. It calms me down to hear you say it."

Suddenly, we hear a cry from another bed. "Nurse!"

"Someone will go to him," she says, handing me more pamphlets about heart disease, heart healthy diets, and cardiac rehabilitation programs.

"Nurse!" the voice calls out again from a stretcher behind a closed curtain. A cardiac monitor goes off. It could be nothing or something, but Nurse Louellen goes to the nursing station to finish her charting. Sitting there, she keeps glancing at her watch to see when her shift is over. No one is going to the patient.

"Nurse!" the voice calls out again. "I need help."

Nurse Louellen says to another nurse – I can read her lips – "Not my patient."

That phrase should be banned.

The clamp is now off my groin so I get up and hobble over, pushing my IV pole. An old man needs a urinal. He looks at me in surprise and I assure him that I'm a nurse in real life and his nurse is busy. I pull back the covers, position everything in place, and wait for the tinkle in the metal jug. "It's hard lying down, isn't it?" I often say to my male patients. "It's easier for us women."

I think of all the years I've been a nurse and the thousands of patients I've cared for. Why should I stop now? In these few minutes helping that man, I am freed from my worries. As a nurse, I feel powerful and capable; as a patient, I feel weak and vulnerable. Maybe my inner nurse can see me through this. It's time to be that good nurse to myself.

Nurses are notorious for not taking good care of themselves, only others. My long-time colleague Maureen springs to mind. She's an incredibly skilled nurse, but I came upon her one day in the supply room, taping up a raw, irritated poison ivy rash on her arms with the medical equivalent of duct tape. She would never dress a patient's rash without cleaning it first, applying soothing cream and a comfortable, soft bandage, but she didn't do that for herself. Nurses don't offer themselves the same care and attention we offer our patients. It's been said you can't treat yourself, but why not? It will only help me to stay nurse, even to myself. Why should I give it up now, just because I've become a patient? After all, I have used my knowledge and skills to help others, why not myself, too? I would never treat a patient like I've been treating myself! I have always prided myself on being a patient advocate, speaking up for patients, looking out for their best interests. I have always used my words to encourage and give hope, not to scare and create fear, as

I've been doing to myself. What if I decide to treat myself with the same compassion that I have for my patients? If I stay nurse and actively participate in my own care, I won't feel helpless and as if things are being done to me.

As Kevin at camp asked, "What can I do to help myself feel better?" I'll let that question guide me, too. All the ways I've encouraged patients, given hope, and bestowed dignity on others, I will do those very things for myself. I have been so gentle, even loving, with patients; now I will do that for myself. I want to get myself in the state of wanting this surgery. To do this, I need to come over to my side; to move from adversary to partner, from passive victim to strong nurse.

It will take courage to make these changes and to be this way to myself. It will be a choice to be more positive and stop generating endless negative thoughts of all that could go wrong, completely ignoring the fact that mostly things go right. Most people do their jobs properly. Most patients get better.

It's going to take determination and courage to make these changes. Courage takes practice, effort, and *courage* itself. (I will fake it in the meanwhile until it feels real.) Thinking these new thoughts, I feel a lifting of my mood and an upswing in my outlook. It's time to make new choices. I don't want to go into surgery kicking and screaming. I want to want this. I will have to put my whole heart into this project, pun intended.

Two days later, when my kids tumble off the bus from camp. I take them into my arms – Max, who lets me, and Harry, who pulls away. I am out of breath from simply hugging them. At home, they beg me to play basketball on the driveway, as I used to do, but after two dribbles I'm done, panting and short of breath.

"Are we going to get a puppy, Mom?" they ask. We had talked

about getting one this summer, when they got home from camp.

I'm too weak and tired to even answer them, much less entertain the possibility of having a dog in the house and attending to
all that that would entail.

I can't continue like this anymore. I will go forward; I will
choose life.

6

ROCK STAR SURGEON

In my new-found state of nearly nirvana, high on this huge epiphany after the cardiac angiogram, I feel confident I can deal with what's ahead.

Three days after my angiogram, Dr. Drobac calls to tell me he's referred me to a cardiac surgeon. "Dr. Tirone David. Have you heard of him?"

In my world, who hasn't? The surgeon with the movie star name and sexy good looks is a rock star! Having him operate on me would be like having Rembrandt paint my portrait or Mozart compose me a symphony, yet I've ridden with this legend on hospital elevators and waited with him in the line for coffee at Tim Hortons. We have even discussed patients together. And, yes, from time to time I did wonder whether my defective heart would ever be so lucky as to land in his gifted hands. But it will probably take months to get an appointment and I am adamant that I won't ask for special treatment. I want to be treated like everyone else and find out if all the dire reports and criticism I hear in the media and testimony from dissatisfied patients will be true for me. I'm hoping to keep my faith in the health care system and I am curious how it will go for me.

Admittedly, my little sociological "experiment" is biased from the get-go by my insider hospital status and privileged demographics – urban-dwelling, English-speaking, middle class, and well educated – all of which will likely garner me quicker, better care. In theory, Canada's universal health care system provides equitable access and treatment to all, but the reality is that it works more efficiently for those who know how to navigate through it. Yet, despite all the problems and inequities, from what I've seen, most people get what they need. We have it pretty good in Canada.

Two days go by, then three, then a week. How long will it take? I am starting to panic. *This is unreasonable!* Now that I want this surgery, I want it now.

Another day goes by and I'm freaking out. I call Mary to gripe about the excessive wait I've been forced to endure and our under-funded, inefficient health care system. As soon as I hang up the phone the red light is flashing. It's a message from Dr. David's secretary. Would I like to see Dr. David tomorrow?

Of course.

Next, Dear Reader, I did what anyone in my situation would do: I google-stalked him. It soon confirmed what I already knew – that he's one of the top cardiac surgeons in the world. I've also managed to glean some fascinating nuggets about the man. Dr. Tirone David has been appointed Officer of the Order of Canada, the country's highest recognition, for his work and innovations in cardiovascular surgery. Born in Brazil, he worked in Africa with the great physician and humanitarian Albert Schweitzer. As a medical student he practised cutting and sewing on leather shoes, training himself to

use both of his hands equally so as to be able to work on the heart
from any angle and not to waste precious time while the heart is
stopped. He specializes in the aortic valve and invented the David
Procedure, a way to replace the aortic root while sparing the valve.
Patients come from all over the world to be operated on by him.
Yet, in one interview, he laments that in Canada, health care is not
for sale. "It's a pity," he says, "but selling cigarettes, not health
care, is what should be banned." Years ago, he could have gone to
the United States and made millions but chose to stay here and
make a few fewer millions. He espouses the benefits of a healthy
love life, claiming that sex is good exercise.

I hope to get back on that medical regimen one day.

For years, I've heard the buzz about Tirone David's stellar reputation, but if I did have any doubts, I've heard the skinny from the
most reliable sources, the nurses who've worked with him. They
dish about all the doctors and know which surgeons have the lowest
infection rates and complications, whose patients do well, and
who they'd choose for themselves or a family member.

I call Meera, my cv nurse friend. "Tirone David is brilliant, a
genius. He's more than a doctor – he's an artist." Then she said
something I hadn't even thought to be concerned about. "He won't
open you up any farther than necessary. He'll minimize your scar
and close your chest himself, not leave it to a junior. He does that,
especially for women because he knows the importance of cleav-
age," she said.

Who cares about a scar? I want to live!

There's just one thing that my cardiologist mentioned in passing
that does concern me: Dr. David recently broke his arm. He might
not be able to do my surgery.

Before going to the appointment, I put extra effort into preparing myself. Since there's no time for a new wardrobe and an

extreme makeover, I work with what I've got. A new outfit, high heels, and makeup – I'm no femme fatale, but this is as good as it gets.

It's easy for me to find my way to Dr. David's office on the sixth floor, but when I'm at work, not a day goes by when I'm not stopped in the lobby or hallway by a worried-looking patient or lost visitor, a slip of paper in their hand, asking how to get to the X-ray department or where to get a drink of water. Hospitals are labyrinthine and confusing – this one especially. They're like huge jigsaw puzzles with interlocking pieces that are constantly being refigured and rearranged as old wings are torn down and new additions created. A radiology department today becomes a sushi bar tomorrow. The medical records department shrinks to nothing as patient charts go online, freeing up space for new dialysis education classrooms. Overnight, a coffee shop morphs into a patient and family information centre. Over the years, I've watched as this place continues to grow and expand, seemingly in constant flux, always being pushed to the limit of its capacity.

In the beige-hued, no-frills waiting area, I settle in to wait and check out the crowd. One thing I know for sure is that if you talk to anybody in a hospital waiting room, you'll gladly take your thing over theirs. I chat with a single mother of two young kids. She's in end-stage heart failure and only a heart transplant will save her. There's a heavy-set man on an oxygen tank and an Orthodox Jewish couple, he in a black suit and she in drab clothes, who sit off by themselves, praying fervently, both looking pale and unwell – and others.

I sit, thinking about hearts. Not red Valentines or hearts o'gold, nor my own heart for a change, but the thing itself. It's the one part of the body that seems animated. If you have ever seen an open chest, you can see the heart do its work, moving blood. *Pump, swoosh, pump.* They don't call it a muscle for nothing!

To me, the mythology of the heart as an emotional centre doesn't make sense. My brain controls my emotions and the heart seems more of an athlete than a lover. The kidney is also a work-horse — a powerhouse, in fact — but it doesn't get the attention the heart does. There's the strong, silent liver, working modestly behind the scenes, staying away from the limelight. It rarely kicks up a fuss unless pushed to the limit, but when that happens, all hell breaks loose. The liver is every bit as formidable as the work-aholic heart or the mysterious brain, but there aren't as many gala balls to fundraise for it. No offence to gut specialists, pee-pee docs, or skin-heads (gastroenterologists, urologists, dermatologists or plastic surgeons), but their organs don't have the same cachet as the heart. The heart steals the show. Yet, I've seen cardiac surgery and the reality is a technical, cut-and-paste job. It's a mechanical repair of something sophisticated, a simple fix of something complicated.

I recall something else Meera told me about Dr. David. She once attended a lecture he gave and a friend of hers asked if cutting into the heart made him feel like God. It didn't make him feel like God, he said, but made him believe in God. The friend was satisfied with the requisite humility his answer implied. "He knows he's God's servant."

But when you consider what they do on a daily basis, it's understandable why some of these surgeons have a God complex. It's preposterous, presumptuous what they do. They stop the heart so that they can do their work. How certain they have to be to have the nerve to slice into a sleeping person's innocent body! When you think of the challenge of surgery, then add a public who wants everything immediately, will jump on any mistake, and is constantly evaluating their performance – we should be glad that there are enough of them willing to take on this work at all. No wonder some have huge egos, throw tantrums, and act like divas. Inexcusable but understandable.

In the hospital, there's always waiting to be done. I am trying to see waiting as an opportunity to practise staying in the moment and being calm, readying myself for what's ahead. It's a reprieve, a time to rest and breathe. One thing I know about waiting in a hospital, it doesn't mean you're forgotten, though it can feel that way. It's a reminder that others are sicker. I have seen the look of dismay, even fury, on families' faces when I've explained that my delay in getting to them was because I was taking care of someone else. Their look says it all: *Why am I supposed to care about the others? Only my loved one matters.* Yes, but we should care, or at least try to. It's probably too much to ask on an individual basis, but as a society, it's worth considering from time to time. We can't have everything right now. We all need to learn to relax more. I'm still working on this.

The secretary comes out to the waiting room to explain that Dr. David had to attend to an emergency in the operating room but will return shortly.

Waiting is always so much easier when you know the reason.

As I settle in to do more waiting, I overhear conversations on either side of me. One patient recounts horror stories of her surgery – "Oh, the pain, the depression, the constipation!" The other boasts of her quick recovery. "Went home after four days! Nothing to it." I move away from all input, good or bad, and take up a seat beside a husband and wife discussing a book they're reading together about personality types – the Sanguine, the Melancholy, the Phlegmatic, and the Choleric. *Perfect white noise distraction for me.*

Eventually Dr. David arrives and apologizes to us all for the delay. He's ready to see patients. The Orthodox couple stands up. The wife adjusts her long skirt and gives a tug to her wig before going in. She's heavy-set but walks briskly. He's anemically thin and moves sluggishly. I can't tell which of the two is the patient, but seeing how unwell they look is a reminder that it's best to go into surgery in tip-top shape. The fitter, stronger, leaner you are, the fewer the complications, the better the outcome, the faster the recovery.

Next, it's my turn and I follow in as that couple files out, looking a little less gloomy than when they went in.

I defy anyone to describe Dr. David without using the word *distinguished*. In his mid-sixties, with salt-and-pepper hair, he carries himself with the regal bearing of an emperor. Tall and stately, in a crisp, immaculate, long white lab coat over dress shirt and pants, he exudes authority, confidence, and self-value.

We sit in his office, a tiny, utilitarian, windowless room, plain and unadorned; there are no ego walls covered with diplomas, certificates, and awards. There's a desk with a computer, two chairs, and a table upon which there are three items: a plastic life-sized model of the heart, red for the oxygenated vessels and blue for the others, and two small gadgets encased in clear plastic – which I recognize as heart valves. Not one unnecessary item, not even the box of tissues most doctors keep on hand. No tears here. He only offers hope. It's what every patient wants but not every doctor can provide.

On his computer, Dr. David calls up Dr. Morse's summary of my medical history, Dr. Drobac's referral letter, Dr. Sternberg's angiogram – all smoothly integrated on our still-evolving electronic patient record. He glances at each report as it pops up on his computer screen, then turns to me and gets down to business.

"Your valve is severely constricted," he says, pointing out the narrowing of the vessel on the image on the screen, "and your aorta is dilated. The valve has to be replaced with either a tissue or mechanical valve and the aortic with a Dacron graft."

Hearing it spelled out like that, I suddenly realize how much work this means for him. With the need to repair my aorta, as well as to replace the valve, it will be a longer surgery and additional risks due to more "pump time" during which my heart will be stopped and I will be kept alive by the heart bypass machine. He asks about my symptoms and I don't hold back now, telling him about my fatigue, the tightness in my chest, my breathing difficulties, and my lack of stamina.

He gets up and goes out to his secretary to see when he can fit me in.

While he's out of the room, I sneak a peek at my chart, open to the screen of Dr. Drobac's report to him. "Thank you for seeing this pleasant, mildly overweight 49-year-old mother of two . . ." it starts out. I guess it's a better description than "interesting case," considerably more optimistic than what one doctor wrote recently in a patient's chart: "A puzzling story that started with a constellation of unfortunate events," and believe me, no one wants to be described as having an oddball condition, known by the nickname of "fascinoma." I'm just about to scroll down when Dr. David comes back in to tell me his news.

"I want to do your surgery as soon as possible. You are symptomatic and it can't wait."

"When?" I ask.

"You need it sooner rather than later." He pauses. "There's just one problem." He rolls up the sleeve of his lab coat and then his shirt to show me his left arm. "My arm is broken." A recent fracture was not set properly and is causing him pain and reduced mobility. He needs another surgery to have his arm realigned. "I would be pleased to refer you to a colleague."

"But I want you," I say, not the least bit concerned about having a one-armed surgeon. I am taken aback by his humanness. *So he's going to be a patient like me, too!*

"It will have to be next week. After that I will be off for mine."

As soon as possible, please, but does it have to be so soon?

"If I do your surgery, I will be with you every minute in the operating room, and later, I will see you in the ICU, but I won't be there to follow your progress on the floor. My associates will take care of that."

Am I worried that my surgeon won't be available post-operatively? Not a bit. Anyway, when doctors say, "I'll check on you later," what it really means is the floor nurses will monitor you for problems or changes in your condition and do what's necessary or pass along their observations. It's like the phrase "we'll keep you in for obser-vation" is just another way of saying "nursing care," because as old Flo' Nightingale said, in her accurate but limited view of the purpose of the nurse: "The central role of nursing care is observa-tion." Yes, the post-op period is every bit as dangerous as intra-op, but by then I'll be counting on the ICU and then the floor nurses to pick up on any problems. Then there's always the Rapid Response Team that will come if I get into trouble. Most surgeons aren't all that interested in the pre- or post-op phases anyway — only the more exciting intra-operative action. But then I recall another of Meera's comments. "I've seen Dr. David stand at the bedside, watching urine, couting the drops coming out of a patient whose kidneys had taken a hit and was going into renal failure. He cares about every detail."

How many of us inspire that kind of confidence in the way we do our work?

Dr. David explains another decision I must make, the type of valve I want. He's probably given this information to hundreds of patients but goes over it with me now with not a touch of blasé. All in a day's work for him, yet he acknowledges the enormity that this is for me.

My choice is between a mechanical valve made from a metal such as titanium or a tissue valve, taken from the heart of an animal such as a pig, horse, or cow. He lets me hold and look at the samples of each. The mechanical valve may last indefinitely, but I'd have to be on blood thinners in order to prevent clots forming around the valve. It also causes a loud ticking that some people find bothersome. On the other hand, while the natural valve doesn't require anticoagulation, it has a lifespan of only ten to fifteen years. Dr. David doesn't indicate a preference or personal opinion but does add that by the time the tissue valve wears out, it may be possible to replace it by a minimally invasive procedure, through a catheter in my femoral artery, and not require another open-heart surgery.

He hands me documents to read. They are consent forms that give him and his team permission to perform this surgery as well as any emergency procedures that might be necessary, including blood transfusions, a pacemaker, and even resuscitation.

The thought of a blood transfusion puts me in mind of the national blood scandal in the 1980s. It was one of the worst public health disasters in Canadian history. The Canadian Red Cross was guilty of distributing blood that hadn't been adequately screened for some infectious diseases. Many units of blood, unknowingly tainted with the hepatitis C or HIV viruses, were given to patients. Thousands of people became infected. But now I try to replace thoughts of that horrific episode with my knowledge of all the measures that have been taken and are now solidly in place to ensure that the blood supply is clean and safe.

Then there's the other, more common problem associated with

blood – the perennial shortage. A famous hospital legend has it
that once, when a patient suffered massive blood loss in the operating room, Dr. David ordered everyone around the table to donate
blood to replenish the blood bank. What if I need a transfusion?
Will there be enough for me? There's no time to store my own.

I return to reading the "informed consent" document. It
demands a true understanding of all risks and benefits, but I often
wonder if most patients get this. If they did, perhaps there might
not be as much blame going around in hospitals as there often
seems to be. "No one told me this could happen," I've heard
patients or their families say when complications happen or things
go wrong. "Oh, maybe they told me, but I was too stressed and
didn't take it all in," they admit. I pull a pen out of my purse to sign
on the dotted line, but again I stop short. Recently, I took care of
a thirty-one-year-old man who came in to the hospital to have a
mitral valve replacement and had a massive cardiac arrest on the
table. He was too ill to undergo the valve replacement and ended
up needing a double lung and a heart transplant. From what I hear,
he's never completely recovered. He doesn't grasp that he's had a
transplant, yet he knows he's not at home with his family. I push his
tragic story out of my mind – it's so rare – and sign the documents.

Now seems like a good time to reprise my chorus, which is
beginning to sound, even to me, like a broken record.

"I want you to know . . ." I start off strong, but my voice drops
down low as if I'm about to say something forbidden. It feels that
way but I continue on with my urgent message. "If something happens and . . . if I become irreversibly brain-damaged . . . or if it
doesn't look like I'm going to make it, please . . . don't prolong my
life endlessly on life support . . ."

Why does it feel so radical, so subversive even, to discuss death?
I struggle for the right tone and the proper words to express these

things yet, I should know how to do this! I've been thinking about
it for years.

"That's not going to happen," he says curtly, making a dismissive
gesture with his unbroken arm. "I'm going to fix your heart. You're
going to feel better than ever."

I've insulted him! I didn't mean to impugn his ability, but surely
even he has lost patients before? Perhaps none died because of
anything he did or didn't do, but he knows what can happen. It's
obvious he doesn't wish to entertain further discussion of this
topic, so I drop it and we chat briefly about his work. He shares his
frustration that his injury prevents him from operating. "There
are so many more lives I could be saving."

His gift weighs heavily on him. *Does this guy ever take a vacation?*

Susan, Dr. David's secretary, comes over to tell me she'll call me
in few days to tell me if he can fit me in next week. If not, he will
refer me to another surgeon. This situation reminds me of when I
was a week overdue in my first pregnancy and my obstetrician
wanted to induce labour because of my cardiac problem. I became
suddenly superstitious, reluctant to tamper with fate. I couldn't
have the baby shower my friends wanted to throw for me until after
the baby was born and I certainly couldn't bring myself to book an
appointment for the birth. What if I made the baby a Libra when he
was supposed to be a Virgo? I don't like to mess with the stars! My
doctor wisely knew how to deal with my concern. "It's already been
decided," he said with a glance heavenward, alleviating me of any
earthly interference. I agreed to book my delivery date.

Dr. David accompanies me out to the waiting room and as I'm
leaving he does something that catches me off guard. He puts out
his hand and takes mine. Many surgeons refuse to shake hands to
avoid picking up an infection or having someone crunch their
bones, yet this gesture means so much to the person entrusting

his or her life to you. (Once, I went to a lawyer who wouldn't shake my hand because he knew I took care of HIV-positive patients. I never went back to him.) I appreciate this handshake. It seals the pact of trust. *Now your problem becomes ours. We are partners and will face it together.*

As I'm about to leave Dr. David's office, as usual, my curiosity gets the better of me and I can't resist one last question.

"Tell me. The Orthodox couple, how do they feel about a pig valve?"

He merely smiles at my question, but I know the answer. To an Orthodox jew, anything is permissible if it is to save a life – even something as unkosher as a pig.

Before heading home, I sit in the bustling lobby, sipping a cup of coffee, immersed in my thoughts. To some, it may seem overly dramatic and extreme to plan my "advance directives" about my end-of-life care. Certainly no one wants to have these difficult conversations, but the thing is, I have seen what happens if you don't: it falls to your (mostly) well-meaning families to speak on your behalf. At best, they can only guess. They each know you through their own, personal perspectives. I have been at bedsides where warring factions stood on opposite sides of the patient, each pulling in their own direction, both sides claiming to know the person best. What I do when this happens is position myself as close as possible to the patient, or at the foot of the bed, trying to show with my body that I am not aligned with either side, only with the patient. Sometimes when there is so much conflict without resolution or where there is no family or "next of kin" – such sad words – to speak on behalf of the patient, a public guardian, a complete stranger who does not know the patient at all, intercedes to help make these crucial decisions about instituting, prolonging, or withdrawing treatment for a person by email, fax, or telephone.

The crux of the problem is that we don't know our ICU patients' wishes. Most of them are far too ill to express themselves. I often look down at them, lying there unconscious, and search for signs that would reveal their wishes. I wish I could ask them, *What do you have to say about what we are doing to you? Do you want this? Should we continue? Please tell us!*

I can't deny the long-held conviction that I have in far too many situations that if they were able to speak, many would refuse to have done to them what we are doing. I can almost imagine their voices:

Let me outta here.

Stop torturing me.

Please just keep me comfortable. Let me go in peace.

For years I had my own opinions but never let them affect my patient care. But it was causing me so much distress that I had to find a way to come to terms with these situations or I was going to have to leave the ICU. Eventually, I reached a turning point with the realization that my job is to carry out my patients' wishes – if only we knew them! (I'll do just about anything a patient wants, unless it's harmful or illegal, but even that's debatable. Have I ever given a cigarette to a patient dying of lung cancer? Of course I have! Isn't this "patient-centred care"?)

I have worked with doctors whose views differ from my more liberal ones. One in particular vehemently opposed this interpretation of patient-centred care.

"I have to act according to my moral code," he told me once. "I have to do what *I* believe is right for my patients as their physician."

"Even if it differs from what they want?"

"Yes. I have studied long and hard to do what I am trained to do, and choosing life is always the right thing. There is no situation when I would not do everything I could to save a life." He did not believe in ever discontinuing active treatment or withdrawing life support. "How could I deny every medication, dialysis, full resuscitation, or life support to a patient? That would be murder!"

"What if the patient told you they didn't want any more?"

"It's a symptom of depression or psychosis. I would call for a psych consult."

"And if it was concluded that they were competent to make this decision?"

"Someone who is mentally competent would not want to die. It goes against everything I believe in as a doctor and I won't offer it. They'll have to find another doctor. Death is the enemy and we have to fight it with everything we've got."

We left it at that. I am happy to disagree but wary of such certainty – of any position – especially when it comes to these matters. Sometimes, lack of resolution makes more sense to me than "answers" to these questions.

But I continually return to the question that obsesses me. What do our patients want? The few times they have documented their wishes, or have been able to express their opinions to us themselves, are so singular that they stand out in my mind.

There was Mrs. Summer, a seventy-year-old woman who had been a patient in the ICU for almost a year. Chronically ill with a multitude of medical problems that affected every body system, she lived on a ventilator, dependent on it for every breath, and showing no signs of ever being able to wean off of it. Mrs. Summer was able to tell us that she did not want to continue living this way. She asked for treatment to be stopped and to be kept comfortable. Many days passed during which specialists of all kinds came to her bedside to determine if she was of sound mind and not merely temporarily discouraged. It was decided that she was indeed capable of making this fateful decision. When she was ready, quietly, slowly, surrounded by her family, life support was stopped and she was kept comfortable while she died. Sad? Strangely, I didn't find it so. It is profoundly satisfying to help a patient achieve her or his goal to die in comfort and dignity.

Another occasion when we heard directly from the patient herself was not as peaceful. A patient with pulmonary hypertension, a serious lung condition, grabbed my arm and told us she wanted us to do everything to save her life. Even as she was gasping what turned out to be her last breaths, she made sure to tell me her wishes for the guardianship for her young daughter. A lawyer was on his way to document these directives, but I doubted he would make it in time so I sat beside her and wrote down everything she said verbatim. "Don't let my sister adopt my child. She is evil. She'll abuse her and make my daughter her slave." She begged me to make sure that wouldn't happen, but all I could promise was to record her wishes in her own words. I had no way of finding out what happened, but at least her wishes were documented.

A much more common scenario is that of an eighty-eight-year-old woman who is currently in the ICU in a vegetative coma after massive strokes and seizures. She is being kept alive on life support because once, many years ago, she and her husband visited a nursing home and she casually remarked in passing about the residents there: "Well, at least they are alive." From that one-time, offhand statement, her husband has concluded that she wants to be kept alive on life support.

As for me, I have done due diligence, telling my doctors and most importantly I have spoken with my family doctor, Dr. Janet Morse. She knows my wishes. Now, before leaving the hospital, I have one last stop. I need to speak to one of the ICU experts. I want to be saved only if it is possible to do so and there are certain doctors I trust to know the difference: Dr. Laura Hawryluck is one of them. It takes experience, wisdom, and discernment, all of which she has in abundance. I've known "our" Dr. Laura for years. Friend and colleague, she's brilliant, kind, and modest, not to mention incredibly chic with her stylish clothes and great vintage jewellery. When I catch her for a moment in the ICU, she's busy but takes a moment to sit with me in the conference room, a big glassed-in area near the nursing station we called "the fishbowl." It is a public place, but we're alone for this conversation. She listens and nods and agrees to be available if I need her. She promises to check up on me in the ICU.

For years I've complained that people need to discuss these matters when they are well and able to consider them rationally, but it's no wonder that most people don't. It's taken open-heart surgery to make me face them myself.

It's time to go home. I look at my watch. I'd been at the hospital most of the afternoon, more than an hour in Dr. David's office alone. Every patient wants – and deserves – generous time with their doctor. If it means waiting for our turn, so be it. From what I've seen and know of him, he treats every patient with the same unrushed attention. And he didn't notice my lacy black blouse or hip jean jacket, nor did he actually examine me. He's only inter-ested in the heart he can see and touch, the first-hand heart, not second-hand on a computer screen or listening to it at the far end of a stethoscope. *Why read a translation of a book written in your native language? Why kiss the bride through the veil?* my father would say. When my heart is in Dr. David's hands, he'll know what to do.

All I have to do is show up and he will fix it.

7

HOW TELLING

It's time to tell my children and the rest of my family and friends. I guess I needed to think it through first and come to terms with it by myself. My family is small — just my brothers and their wives — but we have a wide circle of friends. Vanessa makes it easy for me, showing only concern without a speck of begrudging that my heart defect is fixable and Steven's wasn't. I beg her not to tell her kids to whom I'm very close, but she scoffs at that idea.

"Of course I'll tell them. I don't like secrets," she says.

With my friend Joy, there are some minor grievances lingering between us over long-forgotten matters, but now with this, we are reminded of what's really important, and we let them go.

"I'll visit you in the ICU," she says.

"I'd rather you come afterward, when I'm at home," I tell her. I'm not sure yet how I feel about people visiting me in the ICU.

I called Robyn, a few days ago. Friends since we were ten, at school, Robyn was the pretty and popular one and I was, well, *not,* but that's never mattered. In her family, there are six daughters and I swell with pride when her parents, Dr. Bob and Norah Sheppard, refer to me as their seventh. They "adopted" me during my miserable adolescence when I wanted a different family than the one I had. After all these years, Robyn is every bit as beautiful, with her completely natural, unmade-up looks. Even though we live far apart (she's in British Columbia) and don't see each other much, we know every detail of each other's lives and couldn't be closer or more in tune with one another.

"Remember that day when we were hiking on Pulpit Rock?" I started off, falsely upbeat and dispensing with greetings as we always do. She remembered it better than I did; what happened up there scared her more than me. When I said the words *open-heart surgery,* she gasped, but I continued on, explaining in clinical detail what's involved, underplaying my fears. I could tell Robyn was baffled; she couldn't read me. It was unlike me to be so unemotional, so preternaturally calm. But I've had time to get used to this idea and work toward this state of acceptance; she's hearing the news for the first time. She probed deeper, wanting to know how I'm *really* feeling. "Is there something you're not telling me, Til?"

"Only that anything could happen. I believe it'll go well, but you never know ..."

"Are you having a premonition?" Robyn's in touch with the metaphysical.

"No," I assured her and we fall silent for a few long minutes. Odd, but in our forty-year friendship, we've never been at a loss for words until now. I'm afraid she might cry, so I rush to get off the phone quickly. "We'll talk soon," I promised, thinking how love has a way of reminding you of all you stand to lose.

Now as I tell other friends, they react with surprise and concern. Since no one knew I had a heart problem, this comes completely out of the blue. It shocks them.

"How terrible! That's so scary!" they say. *Could this happen to me? I see them wondering. What are the symptoms? How do you know if you have this problem?* We are all at the stage in life when it's beginning to dawn on us that we won't be around forever. Having kids reminds you of that and so does heart surgery. Their worry burdens me and makes me feel guilty for having caused it. I'm used to making things better for people, not worse. Some friends nervously regale me their own health problems and those of their relatives, or share their hospital horror stories. I reassure them of my good prognosis, and tell them a few medical jokes. I attempt to lighten up and change the subject, but it's not easy now, with this news out there.

One friend asks if I've told our rabbi, but I don't believe in turning to religion at a time of illness or crisis. It seems false to me. But I'm just as superstitious in my own way. I even have a phobia about prayers, thinking they'll jinx me. For example, I never say, "Have a safe trip" or "Be well" because I can't bear to think that a trip, or you, could be other than safe or well. On the other hand, it's just something people say. It's never been a stretch for me to believe in things unseen or unproven, and yes, I do believe in God and feel a desire to pray, but it seems undeserved and hypocritical to start now. Besides, if I was going to pray, I'd do it in out in nature somewhere, where I can feel the presence of God, not sitting in a noisy, crowded synagogue. *How's this, God? Can we cut a deal? If I make it, I will start going to synagogue – as well as every church, temple, and mosque.* Yes, I'll join any group that will accept me and that has good music.

Every since my angiogram three weeks ago, I've had a strong sense of taking charge of my patient journey. I have been preparing

myself for this event like an athlete in training for the Olympics.
I'm taking excellent care of myself, getting lots of rest, eating
well, meditating, breathing, and reminding myself to smile,
laugh, and be cheerful, especially in front of my kids. I carefully
select the Internet information I expose myself to (nothing scary
or upsetting) and am highly selective about the company I keep,
allowing around me only those who are calm, balanced, and positive. The words people say and the energy they bring affect me as
strongly as medications and I take care to titrate the dosages carefully, exactly like I would give a drug in the ICU, one that goes
straight into the circulation.

"Stop trying to direct everything," Ivan says. "You've become a
control freak."

"Some people make it harder for me. I don't want them around
me."

"They don't mean to. They only want to help. People have a right
to react however they wish."

"But if they are anxious or negative or worried, it affects me." I
see his skeptical expression. "I'm talking on a molecular level," I
insist. He shakes his head. None of this makes any sense to him
and only seems like I'm being difficult and ungrateful. As always,
he's maddeningly sensible, but I'm the one in charge and I'm
doing this my way! For now, I've put the kibosh on pity parties,
fear fests, and worry warts. I'm in survival mode and have decided
that what I need is to be around people who are strong, who believe
I can do this, who will let me express my fears, listen, but then
bolster me up. I want to be around only those with a healing,
hopeful outlook. That description sounds like nurses. It's time to
tell them.

One thing that is strange and troublesome is that Robyn hasn't
called back since that phone call over a week ago. It's so unlike her

to avoid or ignore me. I waver between curious and furious. Maybe she didn't hear me correctly? Is it possible she doesn't get it?

There's something else I have to do before my surgery. It was Monday when I saw Dr. David, it's now Wednesday and I could be called for surgery any day. There's not enough time to consult with a lawyer so I sit down to document my wishes about my care in my own words. It's not an easy thing to do. No wonder most people don't do this. How to cover all exigencies and leave no ambiguity? I've heard families argue over the meaning of words such as *reasonable* or *chance* or *recovery*. As one family member put it, "Even a 1 per cent chance is better than 0 per cent. I am holding out for that miracle." Ultimately, whatever I write or say, it will be up for interpretation by the people caring for me, most importantly Ivan, who will be the one to speak on my behalf if I am unable to do so. There's just one problem with that and it has to do with a dog.

Twenty years ago, just before we got married, we adopted a puppy from an animal shelter. A black and white terrier-poodle mix – so cute. The other dogs were barking madly and he was quiet. We named him Rambo, enjoying the joke of such a fierce name for such a docile puppy. Soon after we got him home, Rambo found his voice. He barked at his shadow, his reflection in the mirror, at the ringing of the telephone, and, of course, at the person who delivered the mail. (Question: Why do dogs bark at the mail carrier? Answer: Because it works.)

Rambo barked for eighteen years. (We didn't have the Dog Whisperer back then.) He lived well and had a voracious appetite for all the things dogs aren't supposed to eat, like chocolate bars (Kit Kats, especially) pointy, brittle chicken bones, and gristle and fat scraped from our plates. He loved beef stew but picked out the mushrooms and made a pile of them on the side of his bowl. "I don't know what you're feeding him," the veterinarian said, "but keep it up."

Rambo was a dog's dog; indifferent to our affection, he enjoyed only the company of other dogs. Whenever the front door opened, he'd make a mad dash for freedom, as if busting out of jail. He was always fleeing our home for refuge elsewhere, once at the local high school a few blocks away.

At fifteen he began to slow down. (Afterall, he was really 105 dog-years old!) At night he would fall down the stairs. Lying in bed, Ivan and I listened to him, bump, bump, bump.

"He's blind," Ivan said. "He can't see the stairs. We should take him to the vet."

Why? To be fitted for glasses? How would he read the eye chart?

At sixteen, Rambo went deaf, but it didn't make a difference to us since he never came when he was called anyway. He was the Helen Keller of dogs, blind and deaf, brave and stalwart—though not mute.

At seventeen, tumours sprouted on his legs, back, tail, and penis. He limped and hobbled, his back legs gave out. Yet he kept trying to drag himself to the door, to make a bid for freedom whenever possible.

At eighteen, he was incontinent — all over the house — but Ivan felt it would be undignified for him to wear a diaper. Rambo slept all the time, waking up only for his food. "See, he still has an appetite," Ivan said, not the least bit concerned that he threw up all his food after each meal. Ivan loved Rambo completely and unconditionally, and that was that. To Ivan, love means never stopping love or giving up.

This is what families say. They can't let go because of love.

I hope no one loves me this much, ICU nurses often say to one another.

I loved Rambo, too, perhaps not as much or as well, but in a way that allowed me to let him go. When the time came and he was drawing his last breaths, Ivan laid Rambo on a cushion and brought him to me. "Goodbye, Rambo," I said, patting his furry head (Rambo's, not Ivan's).

We didn't put Rambo on life support, nor did we resuscitate him (though if he'd gone into cardiac arrest I'm sure Ivan wouldn't have hesitated to perform "mouth to snout"), but we didn't do anything to ease his discomfort either. The point is, I don't want to linger like this if I become incapacitated like that, out of control of my body, or in obvious pain. *Please, do the kindest thing and ease my suffering!* Can I count on Ivan to represent my wishes?

If I'm on prolonged life support and it's not looking good, my family will be asked to consider what was important to me. "What was Tilda like?" they will be asked. "What were her goals and values?"

There are certain phrases families always say about their loved one when they're considering what steps to take in their care, and my family will probably say something similar about me, too. One is, "Oh, Tilda – she loved life."

Yes, I do, but on my own terms. I do love life, but not at any cost, not without condition. I love life, but I'm not prepared to compromise. I want to live, not merely exist. I don't want to live if I can't take care of myself and my family, if I have to be taken care of by others. Yes, I believe in the sanctity of life, but even more, I believe in the meaning of life— according to my definition of it, for me. If I lose my mind or my independence, let me go!

The other thing families say and mine will likely say, too: "That Tilda, what a fighter!"

"Tilda never gave up. She wasn't a quitter."

Oh, yes I did, yes I was. I don't take on futile battles or ones that I don't believe in. And I don't want to be kept alive only to exist or to be a burden on my family.

Many nurses feel as I do. Maybe it's because we see our patients' suffering up close and personal. We are the closest witnesses to exactly what they go through. We feel tormented when we prolong and increase that suffering by engaging in futile treatments. We definitely don't want that for ourselves. The irony here being that most nurses say they would refuse many of the very treatments that our patients are receiving. I have heard so many nurses express these sentiments that it would be interesting to conduct a survey of nurses' own end-of-life wishes and compare them with a control group drawn from the public. I have my hypothesis of the results; what's yours?

There are other matters we should all consider – not just those of us facing major surgery – such as organ donation. I need to sign a consent form, but more importantly I must tell Ivan my wishes. Families can override patients' documented decisions. They get to decide because once you're dead, you don't own anything, much less your body.

Power of attorney can be for finances and/or for carrying out wishes about care and treatment, which reminds me of my father's fondness for an old Jack Benny joke about a robbery. (Warning: You may only find his joke funny if you're approaching fifty or about to undergo major surgery.)

A guy is walking home at night and hears footsteps behind him. A voice says, "Don't move. This is a stickup. Your money or your life."

The guy pauses.

The robber repeats his threat. "Your money or your life, mister."

"I'm thinking it over," he finally replies.

So, here's another research question I would like to investigate: How well do the hypothetical decisions of substitute decision-makers (SDMs) correlate with those of the patients who have appointed them? "In Scenario X, would the patient want to have a feeding tube?" or in "Scenario Y, would the patient want to be intubated or prefer to have comfort measures only?" How well do the SDMs know the patients' wishes? It'll be a macabre twist on the old *Newlywed Game,* where spouses are tested on their knowledge of the other's preferences. "Does she like candy or potato chips?" "What did you do on your first date?" "Who usually initiates sex?" Believe me, the results of my study would be every bit as fateful!

Next, I call the members of Laura's Line and tell them, one by one. They promise to check up on me and visit me when I'm home. "Do you remember Rambo?" I ask Laura.

"Of course! How could I ever forget?"she says and immediately knows exactly why I ask. "Don't worry, we won't let Ivan 'Rambo' you. When he goes out to put coins in the parking meter, we'll pull the plug on you."

Laura knows how to cheer me up.

Frances knew Rambo, too. "Remember the day they called from school to say, 'We have Rambo here, in the principal's office?'"

Yes, they remember it all, even the mini euthanasia kit they prepared for me, though I never could bring myself to use it. (Hot shots – they wouldn't have had the guts to do it either.)

It's time to have this discussion with Ivan. In the ICU, when the family and the team gather to discuss a patient's plan of treatment, it's these conversations that become more meaningful and persuasive than any paperwork or legal documents. When we're all standing at the patient's bedsides, trying to figure out what to do, no one has ever pored over the clauses in a living will to find answers, but many families have been asked, "Did you ever have a talk with her about these matters?" or "What would he have wanted?" I want Ivan to be able to say, "You know what? Just before she went into surgery, we had a conversation and this is what she said . . ."

"Ivan," I say when he gets home from work. "There's something I have to tell you."

"What?" he asks, tired and distracted.

Oh dear, it's probably not the best time to talk about this, but I'm down to the wire here – my surgery will likely be next week.

"If something happens to me during or after the surgery –"

"Oh, not this again," he groans in exasperation, covering his eyes. "Do we have to go over this again?"

I guess I may have mentioned this topic before, but doesn't it bear repeating now?

"Please listen to me. I need to say this."

"Can't you be more optimistic? You're going to be just fine."

"Probably, but just in case . . . if I don't, you know, well, make it . . . What I mean is, that if my time is up, let me go in peace."

"You are not going to die. Haven't your doctors said you're going to do well?"

"Anything's possible. It's major surgery."

"We could all die, at any time. What's your point?"

"That's my point! You read the newspaper. You watch TV. You sell life insurance. You know what can happen. Everyone should have this conversation, not just before surgery. People write wills for their money and jewellery, but this is way more important. Everyone should be having this discussion with their loved ones. Maybe it should even be a law! We all have to prepare ourselves and each other."

"Why don't you prepare yourself by being more positive?"

Oh, the tyranny of the Positivity Police! "Look on the bright side," they're always saying. The "glass is half full" proponents. This is not the way I cope with life. I have to take my time to feel bad about what's happening, then, knowing what I know, make a conscious choice to be positive.

"You'd have given up on Christopher Reeve and look at all he managed to accomplish, even as a quadraplegic."

"But he was able to speak for himself and state what he wanted and he chose to live, even though he knew he would need around-the-clock nursing care. I'm not as brave as that. I respect that choice, but it's not what I want for myself."

"Why not? Isn't it better to be alive than dead? To be here for your kids than not?"

"To me it isn't, not if I can't take care of them or, even worse, if they have to take care of me. Please let me go before it gets to that point – don't you dare let me linger around like Rambo!"

"Is this about Rambo or you?" he asks in exasperation.

I see I've touched a nerve, so I keep it to my own situation. "You need to know my wishes so that you can speak on my behalf. Now you don't have to worry about it because you know them."

You should really be thanking me.

In the evening, we take the kids out to a local sports bar restaurant for dinner and as we wait for our food to arrive, I figure it's time to tell them. (Just yesterday, Harry asked again about a puppy. "Not now," I'd said tersely without offering an explanation.) A TV set is suspended up above their heads, facing them. On the split-screen their eyes flit from a tennis match to a soccer game. At the same time, they've made the tabletop into a hockey rink, with the salt and pepper shakers as goal posts, forks for sticks, and a sugar packet as the puck. Since we more or less have their attention, it seems like a good time to tell them and Ivan starts it off.

"Mom has to go into the hospital. She is going to have surgery on her heart."

Mom's heart! I suddenly realize what it means to them.

Max giggles nervously and looks to his older brother to see how to respond. At first, Harry seems intrigued by this news, then concerned. He's a self-possessed, composed boy at fourteen who is not easy to read.

"Are you worried? Scared?" I ask gently, giving him multiple-choice options and suspect it's "all of the above."

No, he shakes his head and stares at me, unblinking. "I'm never afraid. In a movie, if something is scary, I laugh and then I'm not scared of it."

It's a humbling moment when your child is wiser than you.

But there is something he does want to know, a question I knew he would ask.

"Are you going to die?" His big brown eyes are wide and unflinching. I know he wants the truth.

"I don't think so," I say. "I am confident that it will go well. Many people have had this surgery and come out better than ever." I tell them about the governor of California, the hockey player, and other celebrity heart valve patients. "But nothing is certain and there are always risks. No one knows for sure, but I feel positive." They both deserve an answer they can live with no matter what the outcome. What if my last words turned out to be untrue? Everything I've said might be called into question.

Later, when we get home, they stay outside to play road hockey until it's dark. I stand by the window watching them for a while. I think of all the reasons that I have to pull through this for them. I am the one who looks things up in the dictionary, meets with the teachers, buys all the fancy olives and exotic hot sauces, and what about my perfect pancakes? Do I have any last-minute wisdom to impart to them? Floss your teeth! Return library books on time! Make your beds! During other difficult times I've experienced in my life, whenever I made my bed, that small act started the day with a sense of order.

But even if all does go well, I will be in the hospital for at least four or five days and for the first time since they were born, I will be inaccessible, unreachable to them. Afterward, at home, it will take weeks to recover. I can't bear to think there will be days that I will be of no use to them.

I come in the house and consider other aspects of being a patient. I think of a letter we received in the ICU from a Muslim woman who was coming into the hospital to undergo an elective procedure. She knew she would have a stay in the ICU, so ahead of time she wrote down her wishes about the care she wanted to receive. She asked to be kept physically covered at all times, except for medical purposes, but then only the part of her body being worked upon was to be exposed. Her hair was to be kept covered at all times. If she was to receive nutrition, it should be strictly vegetarian. She asked that her prayer tapes be played for her with ear buds. She wanted no visitors and only her husband to be allowed to see her while she was unconscious. She requested to be cared for only by female nurses and never to be placed in the proximity of male patients. We were able to meet all of these requests, made so much easier because we knew them.

It is astonishing that we don't receive more of such statements. It's a huge problem when we don't know what our patients want. They are not telling us.

It's time to revisit my own views on visiting. As a nurse, I've always been flexible about visiting hours and policies. It's been my way of practising my own brand of patient-centred care long before it became a hospital buzz-word or corporate philosophy. I've had conflicts with other staff and managers who've come down on me when I've allowed family members to visit freely. "We have to be consistent in enforcing the visiting polley," they say. Two visitors at a time. Immediate family only. One person to be appointed spokesperson. No visitors during change of shift. Keep visits short. Overnight stays only if the patient is unstable or dying (sometimes hard to predict). Visitors are to call in first to get permission to enter.

Some of these points are for infection control. Others are for the privacy of other patients or to control noise. There's a rationale behind for each one, but I can't find it in me to dictate to others or to be an enforcer. We do not own our patients; we are not the boss of them. To my way of thinking, my patient is the person in the bed along with all the people who call in, come to visit, or care about that person. There have been many occasions when I've spent more time offering explanations and emotional support to families than to my unconscious patient. I find it hard to limit visitors or their visits and tend to put restrictions on them only when they are rude, abusive, combative, or disturbing the patient – which actually happens more frequently than you might imagine.

Some nurses are not as welcoming to visitors. Admittedly, it is challenging to be around the intense emotions and complicated dynamics that families bring to the bedside. It takes skill and maturity to be able to field the barrage of questions coming at you and at the same time be closely observed while you are doing your work.

There's another reason for restricting visitors that is a sign of our times. The staff's right to work in a secure environment and patients' rights to privacy can be threatened when visiting policy is lax. In the ICU where I work, this is a hotly debated and contentious issue. Some of my colleagues have lobbied to have the ICU locked. They say they don't feel safe, and families coming and going freely is a security risk. "We work at a downtown hospital in a big city," they argue. "It's only a matter of time before something terrible happens." Indeed, over the years we have had angry families and, on rare occasions, hostile, threatening, and even violent ones. Many nurses say they feel vulnerable and unsafe. Recently, members of a street gang tried to surreptitiously whisk away the dead body of one of their members right from an ICU bed. The police were called and the plan was foiled. Another family was so angry about the care their loved one received that they threatened the staff, stalked the nurses in the parking lot, and for months paraded outside the hospital, picketing with placards, naming the doctors and nurses they believe caused their father's death, calling them "angels of death" and "murderers." The nurses in favour of increased security measures also point to a recent tragic case of a nurse in another hospital who was gunned down and killed in the OR by her lover, an anesthesiologist she worked with. But can workplace violence be prevented by beefing up security measures? Couldn't these freak occurrences of violence have happened anyway, and still can happen anywhere?

The issue of security for the ICU remains under debate. Personally, I have never felt unsafe at work, but I probably couldn't work there if I did. I'm pretty "tough." Once, I saw a stranger walking through the halls of the ICU eating a slice of pizza. He wasn't a visitor and seemed like someone who had just wandered in off the street. "Who are you?" I asked him. He told me his name. "What are you doing here?" He grinned. "I'm eating pizza." Bristling, I told him, "This is not a pizza-eating area!" and showed him the door. My friends cheered me on. "You go, girl!" A locked door or security system would not make me feel protected; it would make me more fearful. The only thing that makes me feel safe is to work toward creating a culture of trust where safety can grow. In a healthy public workplace, there is mutual trust between the people that work there and the people we serve. I have experienced it and know it is possible. The problem is, how to get there from here?

Another challenge is the necessity to balance patients' need for quiet and rest with the comfort of being surrounded by familiar faces and voices. There are times when even a well-meaning visitor can be a disturbance. One patient's wife assured me that she'd be keeping an eye on her husband's cardiac monitor and "if his heart rate goes up too much, I'll leave," she promised. Later, when she brought in other visitors, she let me know she was still on duty. "If his blood pressure goes over 150, I'll get rid of 'em." Funny thing was, his blood pressure shot up only when she came in! I assured her that we'd observe him together and if he showed signs of stress from too many visitors, I'd step in.

Seeing the patient means so much to families, especially in the ICU. (I'm not always sure of its benefit to patients, but I'll get back to you on that.) It nearly broke my heart the day a mother thanked me for allowing her to sit at her son's bedside for a long period. As I brought her a chair, she said, "The other nurses have kept me out all day. They made me feel like a nuisance." I was not happy to hear that a parent had been denied access to her critically ill son, but I seriously doubted she'd been prevented from visiting for that long, though it's possible. The point is, that's how it felt to her.

To outsiders, it must seem arbitrary and capricious the way nurses enforce the rules. It shouldn't be this way, but too often it can depend on a nurse's mood, personality, ability to handle stress or communicate with families, or even the whim of the moment. Families resent us for it, too. Out there in the waiting room, they share impressions and rate us – the "good" ones versus the "bad, the "nice" versus the "mean" ones.

I guess we have a bad rep. Riding in the hospital elevator one evening, I heard two visitors grumbling about having been asked to leave at the end of visiting hours.

"So, I'm guessing that G for Ground Floor means 'Get Out!'" one said as he pushed the button.

"Yeah, and L for Lobby really means 'Leave Already!'"

"There should be an S for 'Scram.'"

Do I detect a note of bitterness? There have been times when even I've been pushed to my limit and came down hard on visitors. There was one large, noisy family who walked in and out constantly, poking into other patients' rooms, showing up and wandering in at all hours. I was in the midst of giving an enema to their elderly father when they parted the curtain and peeked in. "Is this a good time for a visit?"

"No! You must call in first! *Please.*" I'd already showed them how to use the intercom in the waiting room and explained the reasons for it.

"Oops, we forgot!" they said, yet showed up again a few minutes later, unannounced. "Do we have to call in? We didn't know we still had to."

"Yes, you do," I insisted, "each time you want to come in."

Later that day, they popped back in when team rounds were taking place. I took them aside and explained again.

"You have to call in first. I've told you already. Patients deserve privacy!"

"We visit a lot. It's because we're Jewish."

"I am too. That's no excuse."

"Can't you make an exception for us?"

"No."

I've never understood people who think rules apply to others, never to them. Later I heard the nickname they gave me: the Nurse Nazi.

As a nurse, I warmly welcome visitors to the ICU, but as a patient, I don't want any. First of all, I'll be unconscious or heavily sedated and won't even know they are there. Second, stretched out on a bed, a bag of urine – or something worse – hanging out of me, I do not want to be on display! Thirdly, please allow me to present myself when I am back on my feet and in repossession of my faculties.

The other thing is many people don't know how to visit a critically ill patient in a way that is helpful to the patient. Why would they? It is a completely unfamiliar environment and they are dealing with their own intense emotions at the same time. Nurses can support them, help them move closer, teach them how to talk with no response expected, and suggest what to say and do that's helpful and calming. I'm quite sure that the voices and faces of family members help to bring patients back to the world, but visitors are only able to do this if they are in control of themselves and are able to serve the patient's needs. Too many times I've seen visitors unintentionally add to the patient's anxiety, worry, or frustration.

Sometimes there's even an innocent voyeurism or desire to take a peek and see for themselves. They are hoping to be reassured, but unfortunately all too often the opposite happens. Unless a nurse takes the time to offer explanations about the ICU and what's happening with the patient and to provide emotional support, it can be an even more upsetting experience than it already is. My advice is that if your visit makes it in any way worse for the patient or yourself (not to mention the nurses!) – stay home. If you do come, it may be helpful to know that your visit is likely harder on you than on the patient, who, hopefully, has been made comfortable and relaxed.

I corner Ivan later in the day. "There's something else I have to tell you," I say and see his expression shift straight into *what now?* "I don't want you to visit me in the ICU."

"Are you crazy? Of course I'll be there."

"Not in the ICU. Visit me afterward, when I make it to the cardiac ward."

"I'm coming. You can't stop me."

"Yes, I can. I have rights."

"You are so selfish! Did it ever occur to you that I might want to be there? That I might need to see you, make sure you're all right?"

No, that hadn't occurred to me, and his words make me cave. "Okay, you can come, but not the kids. I don't want them to see me like that."

"What if they want to be there? It's not just about you."

I am always on the alert when visitors ask to bring children into the ICU. If the patient is able to express a desire to see the child, and that is what the family and the child wants, I work to make that happen in a positive way for all. However, many times I question the benefit to either the child or the patient. If the person gets better, the child may have been traumatized needlessly by seeing the patient unconscious and connected to machines. If the patient dies, that frightening image is the one that will remain indelibly imprinted in the memory.

Once, we held a meeting with a patient's family to discuss withdrawing life support for a young woman who had taken a drug overdose in a suicide attempt. We were doing everything we could to try to save the life she herself tried to end, and we weren't making any progress. The situation was grim. At the meeting, the large, extended family was present. We brought in extra chairs to accommodate all the people who had crowded into the room. Suddenly, I noticed a Polly Pocket doll on the table, then the little girl holding it. *There is a child here. We are discussing the imminent death of her sister. Should she be here?* When I raised it with the family in a whispered aside, they agreed and whisked her away. They were in such a state of shock themselves that they hadn't even thought about the possible effect of hearing this discussion on their child, not to mention the impending death of her older sister as well.

On the other hand, my friend Stephanie recently told me a story that was a real eye-opener. An ICU resident said that when he was a child, his mother had died in an ICU. He was not allowed to see her and never got over the feeling that he had somehow been responsible for her death.

Despite the potential emotional trauma that may be caused in the name of being protective of children, I maintain that my wishes are for my own kids not to visit me while I'm in the ICU, regardless of the outcome.

Ivan has suddenly gotten very busy. Always happiest when there's a plan, he gets down to work. He's sweeping the floors and vacuuming, gathering up the dirty laundry left in piles around the house. He shops for groceries, cooks, and freezes meals. Makes lists of phone numbers of friends and family to call from the hospital.

I've been preparing too. This past week, I went to the dentist for a last-minute cleaning and checkup, as is recommended before any big surgery, but especially cardiac. The mouth is a source of infection and loose teeth can be at risk during intubation. When I explained why I needed to be seen so urgently, with my surgery any day, my dentist accomodates me immediately, and he and his staff look concerned.

"No, it's wonderful. I'm very lucky," I say, pleased to show off my transformation to my new, proactive outlook, my positive frame of mind. I have taken charge of this experience!

In other preparations, I have gone for a complete cardiac pre-op consultation. An anesthesiologist asked about allergies (none) and examined my mouth for false, loose, chipped, or capped teeth prior to intubation (none). Beside him on the countertop was his wooden treasure box filled with "goodies," already drawn up in syringes, that most anesthesiologists keep with them at all times, which will be used in the operating room to put people to sleep and keep them pain-free.

After more blood work and another chest X-ray, I met Marion
McRae, a cardiovascular nurse practitioner. She examined me,
reviewed my test results, and wrote *normal* beside respiratory gastro-intestinal, renal function, respiratory status, and skin condition. Not a perfunctory list; each tick improves the chances of a
successful outcome. Then we discussed my choice of the valve. I've
decided to opt for a natural tissue valve taken from a pig, horse, or
cow, already paying homage in my mind to the animal who will sac-
rifice its life for me. I love all animals, but have a special affinity
with pigs ever since reading *Charlotte's Web,* my all-time favourite
book, about a friendship between a spider and a pig. Not only that,
but I was born in the Chinese Year of the Boar. However, my most
compelling reason for choosing the animal tissue valve is that I'm
realistic enough to know that I won't comply with the diet restrictions, blood testing, or medication regimen required with the
mechanical valve.

To ensure I have all the information to make my choice, Maureen
introduced me to a clinical nurse specialist who specializes in anticoagulation, in case I was still considering the mechanical valve.
She wanted to make sure I knew about home-testing methods
for INR (international normalized ratio that must be kept in check
to keep the blood properly thinned), for ease of testing and anti-
coagulant medications currently under development that will
simplify daily dosing.

But I think I've made the right choice for me.

Next, I met Mindy Madonik, the perfusionist who will operate
the heart-lung bypass machine that will keep my blood flowing
while my heart is stopped. It will be up to her to ensure that my
blood receives adequate oxygen and that carbon dioxide, a waste
product, is removed. She'll make sure that the Ph – the acid-base
balance – of my blood is normal and will give me heparin in precise,

adjusted doses so that I don't develop clots. There's no room for error in Mindy's work. She will be the one to stop my heart and to help it get started again. Maybe if I know all the nitty-gritty details, it won't seem so surreal and impossible to me, so I ask her to lay it on me.

"I inject potassium chloride into the heart's blood supply that goes through the bypass circuit," she explains. "This causes the heart to stop beating. It comes to a halt in diastole, the open, relaxed phase of the heart's cycle. It's the 'lub' after the 'dub.'"

"How does the heart start beating again afterward?"

"I clamp off the potassium chloride infusion and in a few minutes the heart starts beating again. Sometimes the heart needs a shock to get it going again or to return it to normal sinus rhythm."

I hope Mick Jagger will be there, belting out, "Start me up."

More importantly, Mindy will be there. A surgeon's brilliant technique is not enough; it will be up to the perfusionist – along with the rest of the members of the OR team – to get me through this surgery and keep me alive.

Then, after a long day of all these appointments and discussions, I met with Clarence, a heart valve patient who had his surgery two years ago. He's in his eighties, spry and active, walking every day and doing this work of supporting patients at the hospital, alongside other volunteer cardiac patients. He told me how smoothly his surgery went and how much more energetic he's feeling now. "You will too," he promised and offered to be available if I wanted to speak with him afterward during my recovery and rehab phase. I wonder if I would do this kind of work, too. Probably not: I am ready to be a patient but eager to leave it all behind me.

It's been six weeks since Max's earache and in that time I've gathered the information I need, faced my worst fears, put my affairs in order, told my friends and family, made my wishes known, and assembled my team. I have become a professional patient. It's been a lot of work, but now I'm ready.

"Most people don't go to such lengths." Ivan sounds weary.

"Maybe they should."

The next day it's Friday, four days after meeting with Dr. David, and his secretary, Susan, calls. "Would you like to have Dr. David do your surgery on Monday morning?"

"Yes," I say, taking a deep breath. Upon exhalation, I let go of all fear.

8

A SLAB OF MEAT

My surgery is tomorrow.

Yesterday, on Saturday afternoon, I overheard Ivan talking on the phone when I walked into the kitchen. "You can't tell her anything," I heard him say. "She knows it all." He handed me the phone. When I heard Robyn's voice, all disappointment about her not calling me back dissolved.

"I'm coming to be with you," she said, all fired up. "I've got my ticket and I'm leaving for the airport now. You're my best friend and you can't go through this without me. Or maybe it's that I can't go through this without being with you."

"Don't worry, there's no need to come," I assured her. "I'm okay now. I can deal with this. I'm actually looking forward to it. I'm curious to see how this whole thing will turn out. Don't come. The flight is expensive and you have to get ready for your classes."

Robyn is a high-school drama teacher and the school year starts in just two weeks.

"I'm coming. I'll be there in the morning,"
"Okay, but no crying. You have to be strong like a nurse."
"I'll try," she promises.

It's Sunday morning and Ivan has gone to the airport to pick up
Robyn. It's time for me to have one final early morning powwow
with the Bagel Club. I'm coming from home and they're coming
after their night shift. Eric, the owner of the bagel shop, welcomes
us to our "reserved" table, but today we don't debate the merits of
a wood-burning brick oven over an ordinary electric one, or listen
to his explanation of how adding salt to the dough toughens the
texture or why he flips them halfway through baking (so the tops
and the bottoms turn out the same). He places warm bagels on our
plates and pours coffee – "on the house" – for us. Jasna and
Stephanie, who carpool together, haven't arrived yet.

"We'll get to your problem in a minute, Tillie," Janet says to me
as she settles into the bar stool in her spot around our table, which
is to my left, "but first, I have to tell you about last night." She
launches into another true story of saving lives on the ICU Rapid
Response Team. Just after midnight, she was called to the floor see
a woman in her twenties, six weeks pregnant with twins, who went
into a hypertensive crisis, with a blood pressure of 240 over 110.
She was immediately transferred to the ICU and put on an IV medication called Labetalol, which Janet has slyly renamed "La-*bagel*-ol."
During the night the woman became tachycardic and lost consciousness. Her prognosis is uncertain, but the fetuses are still
alive. Luckily for her, Janet and the ICU team got to her in time, initi-
ated treatment, and she now has a much better chance of survival.

Soon, the other two arrive. "I can't stay long," Stephanie warns
as she and Jasna settle into their usual places, Stephanie to my
right and Jasna across the table.

"How was your night?" I ask, wondering what made them so late.

"I refuse to answer that question," Stephanie says but then proceeds to do just that.

"The day nurse called in sick, so we were scrambling to find another nurse because it was not a safe double. Eventually Moira was freed up to take the patient and as I'm out in the hallway, giving her my report, suddenly I smelled something. It was bloody stool — you know that smell, don't you? Unmistakable."

Of course, we nodded. Go on.

"Our gross-out tolerance is definitely higher than the average person's," Jasna interjects quietly as she takes a bite of her bagel and protectively glances around to make sure no one can overhear this conversation.

"Nope! Bloody stool has no affect on our appetites!" Janet says cheerfully, sipping hot chocolate.

". . . so I rushed through my report so I could clean her up. It wasn't a complete surprise because she's a known GI bleed and her platelets are only ten so it was bound to happen at some point . . ."

"That's strange. The same thing happened to me when I took care of her last week, also after a night shift," muses Janet. "I guess she's not a morning person."

". . . her vital signs were stable, so I finished giving my report and then gathered up the cleaning supplies and fresh linen — I couldn't leave her like that. I was just about to go back to her when Mike, who'd been on with me last night, came out from behind the curtain. He'd stayed behind while I'd been giving my report and gave my patient a complete bed bath from head to toe, freshened her up, and then thought ahead to get a doctor's order for a platelet transfusion, which he figured was needed, and sent off the requisition to the blood bank. Isn't that guy the sweetest? He's my new hero!"

"Oh, I can just see him," says Janet, "coming in to town on his white horse, saving the day, so you could get here in time for bagels."

"It's because he's a Buddhist," I say, thinking of the handsome, shaved-headed, ascetic Mike, a long-distance runner, team player, steady worker, and a devoted husband and father to two young daughters. "He told me he tries to practise what the Dalai Lama says, 'Compassion is not a transient emotion but a state of being.' He takes care of nurses as well as his patients."

"All I know is he's a great guy," Stephanie says, brightening, "so I am in a good mood now, but that's why I'm late."

They pick up their knitting projects and turn their attention to me.

"It's time to assign you your passwords," I tell them, revealing a little gimmick I've invented to test my post-op cognitive state for the dreaded "pumphead," a known risk of the bypass machine that can include confusion, depression, and memory loss, though in my case, with my prodigious memory, it might be like losing a few pounds — who would notice?

Janet – Whole Wheat
Stephanie – Sesame
Jasna – Poppyseed

"I want you to test me afterward to see if I remember," I instruct them.

"I hope I remember mine," says Stephanie, knitting a new pair of multicoloured socks. ("How many socks do you need?" I've often asked her, but she always insists she doesn't have the patience for any projects bigger than that.)

Janet looks at me and offers her reflections on surgery as her nimble fingers knit away. "You have to give up the controls for a while. It's like being on a plane. You hand yourself over to the pilot, the technicians, the ground control. You know you can't do any of it yourself."

The prospect of surrendering to this degree was one of the things that scared me the most, but now I'm able to take it in stride, breathe, and let go.

"Yup, when you're lying on that operating table, you're nothing but flesh and bones, a slab of meat," Janet says – and knits – smoothly and unerringly. "Even the Dalai Lama would be a slab of meat on the table, if he was undergoing surgery."

"Isn't he a vegetarian?" Jasna asks with a wink, as she knits slowly and steadily.

Stephanie shakes her head, knitting fast and furious. She points to one of Janet's huge bags full of other craft projects in progress, her daughter's A+ English essay, and assorted low-calorie snacks. "Give it to her now," she motions in my direction.

Janet puts down her knitting and pulls out a sheaf of papers bound together like a patient's chart. "Claire and a bunch of us made this for you last night." The three of them sit back and clicking and clacking away, smiling, while I read.

PATIENT: *Tilda Shalof, RN*

AGE: Whatever it is, she doesn't look it!
SEX: Yes! But please wait until fully recovered.
DIAGNOSIS: Broken Heart
PLAN: Healthy Heart

CLINICAL NOTES
Night Shift: verbal report received, care as follows . . .
1930 –   Good luck with your surgery, Tilda! *Angela R.*

2035 –   You can count on us for leg shaves and chin hair
          plucks! *Liz R.*

2104 –   Patient sitting up in bed asking for bagels. *The
          Bagel Club RNs*

2323 –   Patient asking lots of questions and taking
          notes. Possibly psychotic? *Stephanie B.*

2221 –   Prayers right at ya. *Janice S.*

0001 –   Drugs and Hugs here for you. *Kate M.*

0020 –   Be sure to report back from the other side of the
          bedrails. *Shauna M.*

0030 –   Patient resting comfortably. Good luck, Tilda.
          Gary F.

0051 –   Tilda, our prayers and thoughts are with you.
          God bless. *Jim M.*

0100 –   Come back soon, We need you here! *Cheryl A.*

0200 –   Vital signs stable. Your ticker will be all better
          soon. Love ya! *Belle D.*

0300 –   The Rapid Response Team is on call, day or night,
          for any problems. We'll keep you safe. *Wendy R.*

0415 –   Having a bout of early a.m. stupids and giggles;
          wishing you were here to share in a chocolate
          treat. *Claire T.*

0530 –   Drugs + patient = Happy Nurse. *Cyndi R.*

0615 –   Last turn and fluff and puff of my patient before
          I join you for bagels and then home to recoup.
          Jasna. T.

0715 –   Verbal report given to day RN. Any questions?
          Ask now!

Being cared for by your friends? The comfort it brings is greater
than my embarrassment or need for privacy. And that Claire! – one

of the funniest, wittiest nurses around. It's actually painful to work with her for all the laughter she causes – my belly aches and my jaw gets sore. Once, after coming on a shift as Claire was getting ready to leave, I saw a look of disappointment come over my patient's face. "I know, I know, Claire's a tough act to follow, but you need to rest now," I told him. He was tuckered out from the laughing work-out that Claire had put him through.

"The end of summer is a good time for surgery," Jasna says soothingly. "You're past the July 1 hump with all the interns start-ing out as first-year residents."

"Yeah, if there weren't nurses quietly saving those green asses, there'd probably be more summer mistakes," Janet says with a chuckle.

"And don't be a difficult patient," Stephanie warns me. "Listen to your nurses. Do what they say and don't give them a hard time or else we'll come down there and straighten you out." She looks around the table. "Nurses make the worst patients, don't they? Always meddling and critical. They should know better."

Yes, there are plenty of hospital myths and some contain more than a grain of truth:

- *Doctors let you know they're doctors, but nurses will always hide it.*
- *No one wants to take care of a doctor or a nurse.*
- *Complications always happen to doctors or nurses.*

Once, we told a family of doctors that their father – a radiologist – was in stable condition and there was no imminent crisis. When they asked again later, we repeated that he wasn't in any danger and it would be safe for them to go home. Later, we told them his condi-tion was improving. The family finally went home to rest. During the night, their father unexpectedly arrested and died. *Was it because we dared predict a good outcome about a colleague?* We are more willing to make bad predictions and be wrong than make good ones and be wrong. A nurse will never say, "Quiet shift, so far, isn't it?" or "Everything is going well." According to hospital superstitions, these benedictions will cause all hell to break loose.

Then there's the widespread belief that *doctor and nurse patients get better treatment. We take care of our own.* (This one is probably true, but if so, it begs the question, What are we serving up to the others?) When Dr. M.F.X. Glynn, a world-renowned scientist (famous for his work on the coagulation cascade during cardiac surgery, not to mention his invention of Glynn's Glue, a fibrin adhesive system to help stop bleeding – and for his all-black clothes, sly sense of humour, and love of heavy metal music) and a personal friend to many, was a patient in our ICU, he definitely received preferential treatment. Our nurse manager hand-picked his nurses, assigning him only the best and most experienced ones to care for him.

Janet brings the conversation back to the present. "Tilda, you think you've got problems! My Italian friend has psoriasis, arthritis, and breast cancer. If she didn't have bad luck, she'd have no luck at all! In fact, her name is Fortunata, but she goes by her nickname, Lucky. Think about that! You'll be just fine, Tillie," She bundles up her knitting and shoves it in one of her many overstuffed bags. "Well, gotta run," she says with a wave. "I'm taking my boys to a Westie grooming session."

"But you have to work again tonight. Don't you have to sleep?"

"Later. I can't miss this class! Tootle-loo!"

"One more thing before you go," I say to them. "There's something I need to tell you."

"Please tell me this isn't your DNR speech again," groans Stephanie.

"If I get out of control . . . or start acting weird . . ."

"We'll give you a good slap," says Stephanie, "to bring you around."

"Afterward, we'll tell you the funny things you said," Janet promises and launches into another story about when she had her gall bladder removed and how she pulled off her gown and went completely loopy after a shot of Demerol.

"Don't worry, we won't let you make a fool of yourself," Jasna assures me.

"And another thing . . ." I say.

"What now?" they say in a chorus.

"I know you can't kill me – that would be asking too much – but please don't let them try to save me if I'm not salvageable. You'll know the difference." They look at one another with mock astonishment, rolling their eyes at my exit strategy, but I press on because they know perfectly well what I'm referring to – they would say the same things if the roles were reversed. Goodness knows we've talked about these dire scenarios enough over the years! – and they let me rant. "Another thing, if it is my time to go, I want to die in the hospital. Everyone says they want to die at home, but what for? Think of the mess, the laundry."

"Of course!" they all chime in. We nurses are a sensible lot.

"As for my funeral, burial arrangements, I want you to know that –"

"Enough!" snaps Stephanie. "We've heard enough. I've got to get some sleep. I told you I couldn't stay long." She gets up but stops to look at me suspiciously. "Hey, by the way, where's your notebook? Aren't you writing about this?"

"No. There's nothing to say about it."

"I'm sure you'll find something."

Oh, how I long to be firmly back again on this side, safe with my buddies, laughing at it all! It's a lot better where we get to do the reassuring, not be the ones in need of it. This side is where we can enjoy at least the illusion of safety!

They get up and hug me one by one and even after we pull apart, I swear I can still feel traces of their embraces lingering in my body. It's like those warm currents you suddenly come upon while swimming in a cold lake.

As I drive home, I think it all over: the telling is done and the results are in. Nurses lighten my load. I don't have to *nurse* them. They don't react personally and I don't have to censor myself. They don't try to talk me out of my feelings. They take everything in stride and find a way to normalize it. They believe I can get through this surgery and have managed to convince me of it, too.

And, as bluntly as she expressed it, what Janet said is true. On that table, I will be a slab of meat, a conglomeration of blood, tissues, and vessels. I will be pure biochemistry to the perfusionist, carbon dioxide and oxygen particles to the anesthesiologist. To the OR nurses, I will be vital signs, an incision, a body, and someone's patient assignment. For a time, that's the way it has to be.

Once, I heard on CBC radio about a woman who donated her mother's body to medical school for use as a cadaver. Beside her body she tucked in a letter she'd written about her mother. She wanted the students to know that her mother loved to dance, was an accomplished musician, a loving grandmother. What a clever idea and how meaningful to that daughter, was my first reaction, but then I thought of those students coming upon the letter and struggling to keep their composure. If cutting into a cadaver isn't unnerving already, finding that note would be enough to freak anyone out. Some degree of emotional disengagement is how many of us cope with this work, especially in the early days. The ability to stay open and connected but remain objective and scientific, that's true self-mastery. How many young students have that degree of maturity? Or us, now?

Yes, I'm ready. It's taken a lot of work, but I've brought myself

from worrier to warrior and now I do feel optimistic. I believe I'm
going to make it. But how much harder this would be without my
health care team, my armada of watchers, and my circle of friends
and loving family! How bewildering it would be if I didn't know
this world, its rules, routines, and players as I do! Every patient
deserves to feel this confident, secure, and informed. Every person
needs to be able to trust that they will receive this kind of care.

As I may have mentioned, I don't pray, but suddenly a spon-
taneous prayer comes to me:

If I make it, I will dedicate my life to being a better nurse. I will work
toward ensuring that every patient gets this quality of care. It's what
every human being deserves. No less.

Robyn and I have spent a quiet day together with Ivan and the kids.
Now, it's Sunday evening and time to turn on my computer to watch
a YouTube video of Dr. David performing a valve replacement, the
exact operation he will do on me tomorrow. It's oddly reassuring to
watch his hands carry out this nearly bloodless procedure (a cell-
saver machine vacuums up the spillage and returns it to the patient,
thereby reducing the need for a transfusion). Somehow, it helps to
see the surgery detached from the person under the green sterile
drapes, free of fears and questions.

You don't have to be mother, nurse, or friend. Take a break from all of
that. Just let go and be a slab of meat, Janet whispered into my ear just
before she left.

I pack my bag. There have been many belongings I've come
across in patients' bedside tables and carefully packed "overnight" bags — a lock of hair from a dead infant tucked into a
locket, $100 bills wrapped into a washcloth, and even an Olympic
medal, but practically speaking, you don't need much at all. Of
course, as the old saying goes, when you've got your health,

you've got everything, and when you don't, possessions mean nothing. A million dollars or a diamond ring, neither will help you in the hospital.

Here's what I take: A toothbrush. A flattering photograph of myself – to show them and remind myself who I really am. A Middle Eastern good luck charm called a *hamsa* that has a blue "eye" in the middle. It was given to me by a young man named Boaz, a brave patient who fought many battles and made it home.

"Don't forget your toy, Mom," Max says, bringing me my spirometer, the blue plastic gadget the nurse practitioner gave me to use for my breathing exercises post-op, to prevent atelectasis, which is a collapsed lung. He tries it out himself and Ivan tells him to put it down, it could get dirty, scolding him gently. Max and I have a private giggle – two kids behind Dad's back.

On top of my bag I place my health card. It'll cover my hospital "bills" (don't know what one of those thingamajigs looks like), thanks to Canadian taxpayers, myself one of them.

Max has gone downstairs. I hear him singing "The Final Countdown" – *De-de-doo-doo-doo* – and I have a quiet chuckle at that.

Ivan has made a dinner of potatoes, broccoli, and roast chicken – which gives me an idea. I swoop it away, whisk the platter off to the counter, and pull out a sharp knife from the drawer. Insert into the top of the breastbone of the bird. Slice straight down. Crack open. Flatten. A median sternotomy like the one I will have tomorrow. Robyn and Ivan watch my macabre dissection – Ivan horrified, Robyn somewhat amused – but my twisted little pantomime calms me.

Now, after dinner, I'm NPO – *nil per os* – to allow my stomach to be empty during surgery to prevent aspiration into my lungs. Mary calls and we speak for a few minutes. "God bless you, Tillie," she says before hanging up. From Mary I gladly receive a missive from the divine. I study more codes.

Robyn – Lemon Meringue Pie
Mary – Faith
Vanessa – Picasso
Door to staff lounge – 3601
Medication room – 1011
Password – Rambo
Locker room – 323
Combination lock – 11, 25, 15
Bank PIN – 1234 (isn't everyone's?)

In the bathroom, I remove traces of old nail polish so that they will be able to check my nail beds for perfusion to my extremities. I take a shower and after I dry off, I stand staring into the mirror for one last look at my smooth, unblemished, white chest. Squinting, I imagine the cut that will be there, the bloody trail that the scalpel will make. Another odd idea occurs to me. With a dark red lipstick, I draw an incision down the length of my sternum, so I can get there first and have a hand in transforming myself from wound to window.

I wash the fake lipstick scar off my chest and go outside to watch the kids play basketball on the driveway. I catch each of them and give a quick hug as they rush past me.

"*Hasta la vista, baby,*" I say in my best growly Terminator-Schwarzenegger accent. "I'll be back."

In the morning, I say goodbye to the kids.

"So long, toots," Max calls out and Harry gives a little wave. Ivan drives me and Robyn to the hospital. It's a glorious day, clear and sunny — *so was the morning of 9/11,* I think and force that thought out of my mind, far away.

"You'll be all right," Ivan says, giving me a quick kiss. I hand him my wedding ring, which he takes, showing no trace of the ceremony with which he gave it to me eighteen years ago. Practical as always, he attaches my gold ring to his car keys for safe-keeping and hurries off to work, planning to be back when I wake up from surgery later. Robyn stays with me as I check in through Admitting, where I show my health card and that's it. They're expecting me. I shower with antimicrobial soap and don my hospital gown — my soldier's uniform, as I think of it. I climb onto the stretcher, sit on the edge, and breathe, slowly and deeply. Robyn sits beside me on a chair, her knees close to the bed. She scans my face for clues as to how I'm doing and I try not to take in her nervousness. It's always been like that between us; what she feels, I feel and she experiences my emotions, too. There are few boundaries between us. We mix into each other like water into water or air with air. She reminds me to breathe and I do and she, with me.

"Stop watching me," I tease her. "A nurse observes without the patient knowing."

"Maybe I can learn." She wants to do more but doesn't know what. Being here means so much. One day I will get around to expressing my gratitude, but how do you thank someone for holding your life in place while you go far away?

"Don't worry, Tilska," she says, using her pet name for me, which almost makes me lose it. "I'll fill you in on all the details." She knows I can't bear to miss out any moments of life. "You remind me of my grandfather," Robyn says. "He used to say he wasn't afraid of dying, he just didn't want to miss the news."

I perch at the side of the stretcher with one leg tucked

underneath me, the other leg swinging casually. I'm not ready to lie down, not yet.

"I'm so proud of you, Tilska. You're as calm as if you're sitting on the dock at my parents' cottage," Robyn says, "so relaxed and at ease."

Ah, the wonderful times I've enjoyed at Bob and Norah's summer home situated in the wild majesty of Algonquin Park. I take in the love of those dear friends – like parents to me – and breathe in some of that fresh, clear air.

The anesthesiologist, Pat McNama, arrives and introduces herself. She looks me over and I see what she sees: the way I'm sitting, it looks like I'm missing my leg, like an above-the-knee amputation and she needs to check my circulation, palpate my pedal pulses. "Don't worry," I hasten to tell her, unfolding and straightening it out. "I do have another leg."

"That's so nurse," she says with a laugh, "to see something as I might see it."

Then Dr. David and a nurse appear at the foot of my bed and introduce themselves, saying their names clearly, as if it is the first time we are meeting, though I know them both. The nurse takes my vital signs and measures my oxygen saturation, which is 100 percent. Together with Dr. David they review my latest lab values and test results. They discuss with me the surgery and explain exactly what they are about to do – which artery will be cannulated, which diseased valve will be removed, replaced with the specific type of valve I've chosen. They check with the blood bank to ensure that units of my blood type – A positive – are available in the unlikely event I need a transfusion. They ask me about allergies – none. They ask if I agree to having this surgery performed, which of course I do.

I suddenly realize what this is – it's the famous surgical safety checklist in action! How comforting it is to experience this myself!

I've heard many surgeons say, Why haven't we been doing these basic checks and working as a team all along? It has been proven to reduce complications and errors.

Dr. David asks if I have any questions, which now, finally, I don't. He asks the rest of the team if anyone has any concerns or something to say, to make sure nothing has been missed, before proceeding. He removes a pen from his breast pocket and signs his name right on my chest. X marks the spot.

I'm yours.

A nurse gives me a tiny white pill and I place it under my tongue. It doesn't take long for my world to get small, then smaller. As they wheel me into the OR, I look back, try to give a wave. My vision is blurred, but I see the steel table, draped with green towels, the IV pole where a glass bottle hangs with milky white liquid, which is Propofol, the sweet "Milk of Amnesia" we call it. People are prepping instruments, setting up machines, chatting among themselves.

They drop to a respectful hush when the patient arrives.

The players take their places around the table.

I'm all open heart now.

"We'll take care of you," a nurse says and it's the last thing I hear.

9

HOW NOT TO DIE

"The patient is here from the OR . . . a valve. Where should we put her?"

"That room . . . over there . . ."

"Let's move her onto the bed. One . . . two . . . three . . . lift."

I'm alive! At least I think so . . .

A warm hand in mine. "Hello, Tilda. I am Maria Kirchhoff, your nurse tonight. You're in the Cardiovascular ICU. It's Monday, eight o'clock in the evening. Your surgery is over and it went very well. Give me a nod, if you can hear me . . . good. Can you wiggle your toes? . . . Good. Now, squeeze my hand, the right . . . now the left . . . Good."

I made it — or is this a dream?

"Here, Tilda, hold on to this . . ."

What's this thing? A microphone? Am I supposed to give a speech? Okay, here goes. Ahem . . . I'd like to thank the Academy, my family . . .

"It's your pain pump. Use it whenever you need to. Press it if you have pain."

PRESS . . . *down I go . . . Not a second to waste . . . the show must go on . . .*

"Hi, Tilda. It's Maria, your nurse. It's nine o'clock in the evening, a few hours since your surgery. You're doing well, but we're having a little problem . . . you're bleeding from your chest tubes . . . your blood pressure is low . . . we're concerned . . . want to keep a close eye on you . . . breathing tube in your mouth . . . you can't speak right now . . . let it breathe for you . . . just rest . . . nod your head yes if you hear me. I'm going to let Ivan and Robyn come in to visit in for a few minutes . . ."

Tell them to go away! Let me sleep.

Serious, intelligent, swift, intense, present. Maria will save me!

"Tilda, it's Maria again . . . It's ten-thirty now . . . still blood loss . . . your heart rate is good, seventy-five beats a minute, sinus rhythm . . . blood pressure is a hundred and one over fifty-eight . . ."

I have a blood pressure . . . whoopee! That's a start.

"We're keeping you intubated . . . you're breathing at a good rate of twenty breaths a minute . . . just let the breathing machine help you, try to relax with it . . . your chest sounds clear . . . your blood sugar is up a bit, but I'll keep an eye on that . . ."

Her voice . . . soft, low, and gentle. I am safe in her hands.

"I see you're using your pain pump a lot. Are you still in pain?"

Yes. No. Don't know. Get me outta here! PRESS . . . *and melt into bed.*

Maria, in a different voice, speaking to someone else . . . Who's there?

"I'm worried about her . . . blood loss . . . drained 150 cc of blood from the right pericardial chest tube and 220 cc this hour from the left . . ."

Can I go home now?

"... her blood pressure has dropped down to one hundred systolic, though her mean is still around sixty ... Her hemoglobin is only sixty after one unit of blood ... She's still acidotic with a Ph of 7.34, likely due to bleeding. I'll give her another unit of blood ... She has pain. She's using a lot of narcotic ... urine output is adequate ... she's put out 75 cc this hour ...

What is this thing between my legs? It's a snake! Get it off me!

"That's your foley catheter, Tilda ... for your urine."

Take it out. I don't need it!

"Try not to pull at that ... you might hurt yourself."

"Tilda, it's 11:30 now. You're still in the ICU and you're losing a lot of blood ... hemoglobin is dropping ... given you blood transfusions ... I've called Dr. David at home ..."

I'll be fine. Don't worry about me.

"He's coming in ..."

But he has his own surgery tomorrow. Don't bother him.

"He may have to take you back to the operating room. . . . to see if there is a bleeding vessel or a problem with a suture."

What's wrong? Something must be wrong!

"She's still bleeding ..." *Maria's calm voice, telling someone — who?* "She's put out almost two litres so far ... through all three chest tubes ... blood pressure is down to eighty sytolic ... had to go up on the dopamine ... urine output is good, at 50 cc hourly ..."

"Tilda, it's Dr. David here."

You've come in just for me? Maybe you do love me after all!

"... I'm going to fix this problem ..."

Don't worry about me. How's your arm? How long have I been in here? A year?

"Maria has been trying to stop the bleeding but . . . blood transfusions . . . plasma, too."

I'll be okay . . . You've all been very nice, but I just want to go home.

"Tilda, it's your nurse, Maria. We're giving you more blood transfusions. You're still bleeding from your chest tubes . . . can't find the
cause . . . may be a reaction to the heparin or a problem from the surgery . . . Dr. David may have to take you back to the operating room."

Another voice in the darkness around me. ". . . Could be a coagulo-
pathy . . . what's her INR? Her platelets?"

*Too much garlic, magic mushrooms, Meera told me . . . they can cause
bleeding . . . funny 'shrooms, she said . . . It's funny, but am I laughing
or only thinking I'm laughing?*

"It's high . . . 3.6 . . . Give her two units of plasma . . . her hemoglobin is down to fifty . . . Give her another unit of red cells . . .
that'll make it three units in total."

"See if we can bring her hemoglobin up to at least seventy . . ."

"Her blood pressure is holding, but her heart rate is up to one
hundred and twenty . . . sinus rhythm, no ectopics. . . . she may be
hypovolemic . . . what's her CVP?"

"It's nine milimetres of mercury . . ."

"Give her more volume . . ."

"Tilda, Dr. David here . . . I'm going to manipulate your chest
tubes to try to get the bleeding stopped . . . if I can't, I'm going to
take you back to the operating room and open you up again. . . ."

Haven't I been opened up enough?

". . . there's a ruptured appendix in the OR . . . can't take her back
right now . . ."

"Give her another two units of packed red blood cells and some
fresh frozen plasma, two or three units . . ."

PRESS . . . *Down, down, down I go . . . gone.*

"Tilda, I'm the endocrinology resident, on-call . . . you're having some blood glucose instability . . . Your sugar is too high right now . . . common post-operative complication . . . sometimes happens with the stress of critical illness . . . I'd like your consent to start an insulin infusion . . . Your blood sugar has gone up significantly . . . can have dangerous results . . . a precursor to diabetes . . . lifestyle and diet changes eventually, when you get home, but for now . . . Your nurse will monitor your blood sugar closely and give you insulin as needed . . . Are you in agreement with that plan?"

No, no insulin. I'm not a diabetic! You have the wrong patient. Do you hear me? I can't hear my voice!

"It's important to keep your blood sugar levels under tight control . . . you're a nurse, aren't you? So you probably know all about this, right?"

I certainly do! I wrote a paper "How Sweet It Is! The Nursing Management of Tight Glucose Control During Critical Illness" . . . presented it at a critical care conference . . . Now I'm the subject of the study!

"We're going to start the insulin infusion, okay? . . ."

Sure, whatever you say . . . but I really don't need it.

Maria's calm, serious voice: "I'm concerned about her breathing. Her resp. rate has gone right down . . . She's apneic . . . not breathing enough . . . using the pain pump frequently . . . suppressing her respirations . . . down to six breaths a minute."

I'll breathe, don't worry, I'll breathe, I promise . . . in a minute or two . . . I'll get to it.

PRESS . . . *Down, down, down I plunge into my warm, cozy cave.*

I'm still alive . . . at least I think so . . . fading in and out . . .

"She's not breathing enough."

An unfamiliar voice. Who's this?

"I'm going to lock out her pump. She's giving herself too much narcotic . . . Respirations only ten . . . now six . . ."

The unfamiliar nurse voice.

"She needs Narcan to counteract the narcotic."

No, no Narcan! Bad side-effects. Don't worry, I'll breathe. I promise! Just watch me.

"Her respirations are at five . . . now four . . . a minute . . . She's not breathing enough."

"Breathe, Tilda!"

Okay . . . will do . . . I'll get on to it. Just give me a minute or two . . .

"I'm here, Tilda."

It's Maria, her wings spread over me. From a dark, dense fog, I reach out to her.

Where's my nurse! Do these people have any idea what they're doing? Maria is in cahoots with Dr. David . . . a conspiracy against me . . . Does he love her now? I thought he loved me!

"Tilda. It's Maria. I'm right here."

Her hand in mine. Squeeze.

"How much narcotic has she had?"

"Six milligrams."

Only six? That's not much morphine. Do they think I'm a drug addict?

"What's she getting?"

"Dilaudid."

Oh, six milligrams of dilaudid? That's a whopping dose — fit for an elephant in a zoo. That works! Never mind.

"Good morning, Tilda . . . It's Tuesday morning, seven-thirty . . . your surgery was yesterday. I'm your nurse today . . . My name is Joy Bartley . . . I'll be taking care of you, Tilda . . . be with you all day . . . you're doing much better . . . Maria told me you had a rough night

. . . lost a lot of blood . . . but they got the bleeding stopped without having to take you back to the OR, which is great news . . . Your vital signs are stable . . . you're doing very well. We're going to get that breathing tube out shortly . . . first I'm going to give you a bath . . . freshen you up."

I open my eyes to see my new saviour. Joy . . . a tall, elegant black nurse, strong, smart, capable, encouraging. It's her turn to save me. Her arm on my arm . . . a soothing touch on my forehead. She leans down into my bed to meet me there, touches my shoulders, my forehead, my cheek. Her healing hands all over me. *I'm a baby again, swaddled in warm towels, clean and fresh, like new.*

A tiny ray of sunlight filters through the dungeon window . . . a sweet voice with bright flashes of ruby red at her neck, sapphire blue on her fingers . . . Beautiful bling!

"Tilda, it's Dr. Hawryluck — Laura — from Med-Surg ICU. I promised you I would come and check on you."

There she is, I can see her, bright flashes of colour and singing sounds. Why is she standing so far away?

"I came to see how you're doing. You had a difficult night, but how are you feeling today?"

Shimmering, opalescent mother-of-pearl, shining like moonlight, she's moved in closer.

Love your sparkles! Why are you here again, with your kind face and intelligent hands, tender touch on my arm? Remind me? Chunks of aquamarine, chunks of topaz catch the light on her fingertips . . . Tripping the light fantastic . . . She's elegance and class. I'm lying here, a mess in the bed.

Laura leans down low, whispers into my ear. "Is this all research for you, Tilda? Are you taking notes in there?"

Of course I am! Why are you whispering?

—

"Tilda, it's Nurse Joy here. You're doing well . . . the bleeding has stopped now and your vital signs are stable. I've paged the respiratory therapist to come and extubate you . . . need to be awake enough to breathe on your own . . . are you in there, Tilda?"

Of course I am. I made it! Where did you think I've gone?

Are you feeling okay? I hear you had a lot of pain.

I feel wonderful! The best I've ever felt!

"Hi, Tilda. I'm your respiratory therapist . . . here to remove your breathing tube."

Is it still in? I thought they took that out already.

"There we go. It's out. Give a strong cough . . . And another . . . Good! Your throat might be sore for a while . . . don't forget to use your spirometer and do your deep breathing and coughing exercises so you don't get fluid in your lungs."

Deep breeding and coffee outside? What? When's that happening?

"Tilda, you have a visitor. Your friend Joy is here."

But you're Joy. You're Joy, the nurse, right?

"She wants to see you."

Go away!

"Joy, please wash your hands first and keep your visit short. Tilda's very tired."

No! I said no visitors! Am I still in the ICU?

"Look, Tilda, Joy brought you a box of chocolates."

Please go away . . . but you can leave the chocolates!

"I'll tell her to come back another time."

"Hi, there, dear . . ." Robyn's parents . . . precious faces hover above me, kiss me on the forehead, hold my hand . . . *it's so nice of you to*

*come, but what is this nice lady's name — Cora? Dora? It's Norah! She's
wearing a white blouse, red sweater. It must be July 1. Happy Canada
Day!* I smile at them.

"It's August 26, dear," someone says.

*Don't worry about me . . . I know what's going on. Am I saying these
words or thinking them? I can't tell.*

"Hi there . . ." *My voice is raspy, unrecognizable.*

"Tilda, I'm going to take out the big intravenous and pulmonary
artery catheter from your neck. We used it to measure the pressures in your heart, but everything is normal now and you don't
need it anymore . . . don't worry . . . this may feel a bit strange, but
it doesn't hurt. . . ."

I am completely cared for . . . I let go . . . no pain.

Every time a nurse comes toward me, beside me, around me,
something pleasant happens. A tube is removed, a soothing word,
a touch. I look forward to the voice, the hands. I move toward each
thing that happens and each time, I'm lighter, brighter.

I just might make it.

"Hi, Tilda. It's Christine. I'm your nurse today. I'll be transferring
you to the floor soon. You're doing so well. That's good. Open your
eyes. . . . I'm going to remove your chest tubes . . . first I'll give you
some pain medication . . . doesn't hurt but will be uncomfortable
for a few moments . . . as they're coming out . . ."

*Yes . . . like I'm being eviscerated . . . as a cat pulls out the entrails from
a mouse . . . weird sensation . . . shuddering feeling of being disembow-
elled . . . my guts pulled out . . .*

No, it doesn't hurt, but strange . . .

Nurse Christine Sterpin at my side. Pretty, pink, cheerful, energetic, hopeful . . .

I'm a shipwrecked sailor, swimming toward her safe shore.

"Time to transfer you to the cardiac ward now, Tilda. We're on our way!"

So that was the ICU. *I survived!*

10

FROM VERTICAL TO HORIZONTAL

I open my eyes. At the end of my bed, a sign on the wall:
  Your nurse's name is: Melissa ☺.
  Very good, but what's *my* name?
  How many days have gone by?
  I made it . . . I guess.
  I lift my head up from the pillow . . . barely.
  Brain cells intact . . . more or less.
  "Pleasantly confused" we call it in the biz.

Minutes – or hours? – have passed. Voices buzz at the doorway.
  "Isn't she the one who wrote those books?"
  "Yeah, it's her."
  "I think I'm in one of them."
  Ha, you wish.

—

A nurse – is it Melissa? – arrives. "Here's the call bell." She holds it out to me, but I don't take it. She pins it onto my pillow. I look away. Never! I will have to be *in extremis,* practically dying, before I'll use the call bell. I know what it's like to be summoned like a servant, expected to drop everything, and come running. *On the other hand, how reassuring it is to know that help is at hand.* Nurses hate the call bell. Patients love it but curse it if it doesn't "work": when they push the button and no nurse instantly appears – *poof!* – like magic, a genie in a bottle.

"When I call you, you come!" a patient snarled at me once. I was working on the floor and had five other patients to get to and call bells were ringing one after another. When I finally got to him, he was in a rage, banging on the siderails with his metal urinal.

"You're probably gist sittin' out there on your ass, gabbing with your girlfriends," he said. "You do as I tell you." He ordered me to take away his finished breakfast tray, come back and flip his pillow, then raise, lower, then raise again, his bed in infinitesimal degrees.

Remind me, please, why am I supposed to care about you? Silently, I managed to contain my irritation and did what he asked. I wish I'd told him off – I would now – but back then I thought we were supposed to just take that kind of abuse.

The call bell rests on my pillow. *I dare you,* it taunts me. *Just try me and it's game over, you'll be a patient, helpless and needy.*

I float on a cloud. Sunlight floods the room, warming my eyelids. I open them slowly.

Under anesthesia, you are gone. Where, I don't know, but it's far away. Bits and pieces of the ICU linger – Maria's eyes locked on me, Joy's healing hands on my body, and Christine's positive energy, coaxing me back to life. I was incoherent and disoriented, saying strange things; there was no connection between my thoughts and my words. I thought I was speaking out loud when I wasn't, convinced I was making perfect sense, but I wasn't.

My throat is scratchy from the tube, but I don't have any memory of the sensation of being intubated. How bad could it have been if I don't remember it? Perhaps pain only hurts if you're aware of it? They must have given me sedation for comfort, analgesia for pain, but made sure I was alert and breathing enough to breathe on my own. That takes skill. Who wants to be awake while intubated? Not I. As for discomfort, I had none, but I was using the pain pump repeatedly, going at it like a drug fiend, as if I had no understanding of its use.

I glance down. On my chest is a white, heavy bandage. I touch it lightly. It feels much bigger than it looks. I gaze around the room, but that effort tires me so I close my eyes.

Cheery nurses come in and out, not the least bit concerned about my mumblings or glazed stare – or this huge, new lump on my chest.

"Time to get up," Nurse Melissa says.

Get up? Is she kidding? Is this a joke? Apparently not. "I can't do it," I tell her.

She doesn't take no for an answer and stands facing me, puts her arms on either side of me, under mine, and eases me up to a sitting position. She gives me a moment to catch my breath, then swivels me so that my legs are dangling at the side of the bed.

She looks so young and I feel so old. Does she see only the rumpled, groggy me or the real me?

She turns her head away to cough.

"Are you sick?" I draw back slightly, afraid to get whatever she's got.

"A bad cold. But I'm okay." She lifts me up to stand on my feet. Held there in her arms, I inhale her deeply. *A strong whiff of vanilla and patchouli, a spicy chocolate cake.*

"I have to go to the bathroom." *How am I going to get there?*

"You can walk. I'll help you."

I get up – *oh no, I've wet the bed. Attention, shoppers. Clean up in aisle nine!*

"Don't worry," Melissa says, placing me onto a chair and then quickly changing my sheets. "It happens sometimes after the catheter has been removed. Come, I'll help you to the bathroom."

She expects me to walk there? By myself? Is she nuts?

Slowly, she leads me there and then back, lowering me down on to the chair. "Here are your pain pills." She places them on the table in front of me, then hands me my spirometer for my breathing exercises.

I have to do this. I don't want to get atelectasis. I pick up my "toy," as Max called it, and blow into it. The ball remains at the bottom of the contraption. Why isn't it moving? *It must be broken. Oh, I forgot.* "*Suck, don't blow,*" I've told many patients, realizing only now how lewd that instruction sounds. Once, a patient joked, "After all I've been through and now you're passing me a bong?"

Melissa watches me do a few rounds as she moves toward the door. I'm sure she has a few others like me to get to.

One more inhalation on the spirometer and the ball jumps to the top of the plastic cylinder tube like it's supposed to. That's all for now.

"You're doing great," she calls out before she vanishes.

I'm feeling better. They give you give good drugs here. I like this place.

—

Later – how much later? I have no idea – I walk to the bathroom by myself, wobbly on my feet. It feels like a major accomplishment. I pee into a container, measure my urine, then pencil in the amount to a tally sheet taped inside of my door. I want to be helpful to my nurses, but I wonder if they'll see it that way. Maybe they'd prefer if I were a "regular patient," but it helps me to stay nurse. "The best care is self-care," my friend Nurse Deanna Patricia Bone writes in her book, *Nurse Pat's Practical Guide for Caregivers*. It's my new mantra. I make my way back to the chair, sit and breathe, not for mindfulness, but for oxygen. *I did it!*

Breathing is hard. Something is wrong with my breathing. My heart is racing.

Breaths laboured, SOB – shortness of breath – even at rest. Respiratory rate thirty-six breaths a minute – patient is tachypneic. Heart rate one hundred after moderate activity.

What's wrong with me?

A cluster of doctors stand outside my door reviewing the case – me! They don't seem the least bit concerned with my heart rate or my difficulty breathing. They don't even notice.

"Aortic valve replacement and repair of aortic root," I hear them saying. "Day three post. Had episode of post-operative bleeding... hemoglobin dropped to forty-eight... given plasma and red blood cells... hemoglobin now seventy... Otherwise uneventful."

Yes, a routine case, but *FYI – those are the one's that'll get ya!* You see the same things over and over. This is normal for a post-op valve job, but how to stay alert to the exceptions, the ones who veer from the norm and the subtle signs that trouble is brewing? *I'll keep an eye on it for you.* Sometimes the basic things get missed, like vital signs, for instance.

Relax, let them worry about it; it's their problem now. My breathing is better. No worries.

—

Flashes of the ICU return. Darkness and light, noise and silence, movement and stillness – far away, down a long, deep tunnel. Not unpleasant but strange.

For as long as I live, I will never forget Miriam, a patient from Rwanda. I don't remember her medical problem or much about her, other than her having the worst case of ICU delirium I'd ever seen. She had harrowing hallucinations and just witnessing her going through them was disturbing – I can't imagine what it was like for her. She would be in a deep sleep then suddenly, as if from a shotgun, she'd startle awake, eyes bulging out, finger madly pointing in front of her, at something only she could see, only she could hear. I tried to console her – we all did – but she was unreachable. We tried many different medications to help her but none worked. "What does she see?" I asked her sister one day.

"Her children. She hears their screams. They were murdered in front of her in the village. Then they raped her and left her to die, but she survived."

What was it about the ICU that brought this horror back to her?

"Hi, Tilda, I'm Marion McRae, your nurse practitioner." A tall, attractive woman bends way down to where I lie in the bed to listen to my heart and lungs. She palpates the pulses in my legs and feet. Gently and smoothly, she slides out the pacemaker wires from where they had been placed, inside my heart – weird sensation but not painful – leading out to a pacemaker box hanging on the IV pole.

"How are you feeling?" she asks as she sits down beside me.

"Weak. I have . . . difficulty breathing . . . at times. My heart is racing."

"It's because your hemoglobin is still low, only seventy-one today. You lost a lot of blood after your surgery. You're on iron supplements and your bone marrow will produce more red blood cells, but it takes time. Eventually, you will get your strength back."

Nurse Melissa has returned to take my vital signs, test my blood sugar, and give me more pain meds. I don't see her wash her hands before touching me, but I'm hoping she did before she came in. It's not so easy to ask, from this side, so I let it go. She's a new grad, she tells me, fresh out of school, this is her first job, she says proudly.

I want to reassure her, *You won't always have miserable patients like me. Well, you probably will, lots of them. Please stay in nursing for a while, don't leave us yet, though you might want to lose the perfume!*

I once worked with a nurse who wore a perfume called Opium, which made me nauseous. Another time, a patient's visitor was drenched in Obsession. Within a few minutes, I got a searing migraine and had to go home.

"Here's your lunch, Tilda."

A tray is placed in front of me. What's this? A diabetic meal? This isn't for me! This is a mistake. Only 1,200 calories a day? Who's idea is this?

It's like my father's old joke: the food is terrible and such small portions!

Breathing is difficult. I take a breath and wait breathlessly for the next.

I reach for the call bell — but stop myself.

A nurse I knew had an automatic signature on her emails with the motto "Until the call bell rings . . ." *For whom the bell tolls . . . it tolls for thee.*

"I pushed the call bell a hundred times," a friend's mother once said, recounting her hospital war story after bowel surgery. "I was bleeding to death. I was lying in bed and blood started pouring out of my rectum. I called for help, but no one came. The siderails were up so I couldn't get out of bed, so I scrunched down and slid out the bottom. I wrapped myself in sheets and I held my arm up, the one with the IV. When I got to the nursing station, the nurses laughed and said, "Oh, here comes the Statue of Liberty."

Ouch! Outraged patients have been known to exaggerate their hospital horror stories just a tad, but if this one is even partially true – and it comes from a reliable source – it's horrific.

I've heard of patients who used the call bell and when no one came, they got so frustrated they called 911 from their hospital beds. I've walked through wards where halls are empty, the nursing station vacant, no one was around. *Who's minding the mint?* Where have all the nurses gone? Everyone is busy with someone else. If you happen to see a nurse, she or he is rushing past, distracted, running off somewhere else, to somebody who apparently needs them more than you. A nursing professor told me that when he was a patient, he fainted after a hernia operation. A cleaning staff was mopping the floor and pushed the call bell for help. When no one came, she helped revive him herself.

Melissa pops in. "Do you want to go for a walk, Tilda?"

What am I, a dog? Are we going to the park? "No," I answer curtly.

"You need to walk. It's good for you."

She won't take no for an answer. She stands holding my leash – my IV pole – waiting for me to get up. I guess I'm supposed to be able to do this by myself by now. *Oh snap! This is hard.* Melissa's still not feeling well herself. She's sniffling and congested. Her eyes are bleary. She stands away from me to cough. The prospect of coughing makes my chest ache. Sneezing? Forget about it! What if I get her cold? Will I have the strength to fight it off? "Maybe you should have called in sick?" I ask her.

"They were short-staffed and, besides, I'm casual."

That means she has no sick benefits, but it's no excuse for coming to work and spewing out germs on others. She walks me outside my room and I catch sight of myself in the hallway mirror, my hair going in all directions, pale, hunched over, frail, and dopey-looking, like a zombie. *I'm stoned.* I force myself upright, pretend to be strong.

"Time for your chest X-ray, Tilda, and an echocardiogram." A porter pushes me along in a wheelchair that I have no recollection of getting into. We're rolling down the highway – I mean, *hallway* – at a good clip . . . turning a sharp corner – *wheeeee!* They should put a fake steering wheel on these things to give us patients at least the pretense of control. I am backed into the elevator, not facing the wall. I appreciate that.

Enid, the service elevator operator, cranes her neck to get a look. "I know you!" I nod weakly. "I used to see you like this." Her big arm flaps up and down beside me in a vertical chopping motion. "Now I see you like this!" Her arm slices the air across my chest, flattening the horizon.

After the chest X-ray, I ask the technician, "What are those things?" I point at little squiggles on the black and white picture of my heart, lungs, and ribcage on the computer screen. Little bows that look like twist ties on garbage bags.

"They are the sternal wires to hold your ribcage together,"

Oh. My chest was cracked open – I forgot about that. That's why it hurts to laugh. Good thing nothing's funny.

The radiologist reviews the images of my heart. "It looks good, although it will take time for your heart to recover. But all the cardiac measurements show improvement."

Still, my body feels fragile, cracked into pieces. Will I ever be strong again?

In the afternoon, Mindy, my perfusionist, comes for a visit and brings me a strawberry and banana protein shake from the downstairs juice bar. I sip it slowly. So cool and refreshing. She tells me about the operating room and how quiet it gets when the heart is stopped and the surgeon is sewing. "There was definitely more tension in the room because it was one of our own," she says. "We even talked about your books."

"What, during the surgery?" I look at her in surprise.

"Yes, Dr. David said he read them and liked them. A lot."

"Lucky for me!" *Imagine if he didn't.*

How am I going to thank all of the people who saved my life?

Dear Mindy,
Thanks for stopping my heart and for keeping oxygen flowing to my brain! Thanks also for starting it up again. Have a nice day. Best wishes, Tilda

What about the people who donated blood? Had blood been unavailable or had I not agreed to blood transfusions, I would surely have died.

Marion, the nurse practitioner, comes back and sits with me for a while. She explains that the diabetic diet is to get my blood sugar levels back to normal. They can be unstable post-operatively or with an episode of bleeding. "You're in a pre-diabetic state. It will likely resolve, but you are going to have to watch your diet from now on."

I'm starting to connect the dots. I'm not diabetic yet but could be soon if I don't start taking better care of myself.

As the day wears on, I'm vaguely aware of visitors coming and going and their mild shock at seeing me. But when my gal pals from Laura's Line – Laura herself, Frances, Tracy, and Justine – arrive, they take one look at me and aren't the least bit fazed to see me like this, frail and helpless, sitting there in my faded blue hospital gown. *Maybe it's one I put on a patient myself!* They're wearing bright summer clothes, so animated, full of life, in their usual high spirits, chatting and laughing.

When a nurse comes in to take my blood pressure, Justine nudges her. "Is Tilda giving you a hard time? Put the cuff around her neck instead."

The nurse places the temperature probe in my outer ear canal.

"Why not take it rectally?" Justine suggests ever-so-helpfully, and the others cackle with laughter. "I hear it's more accurate that way. Tell me, is she being a difficult patient? If so, I give you permission to 'go nurse' on her!"

"I thought you were my friend," I complain. "Don't make me laugh. It hurts."

"You're saying some pretty funny things yourself," Frances tells me.

"Yeah, you're a regular sit-down comedian," says Laura.

I can hear myself muttering weird things like my IV "isn't in straight" and something about "tuna fish in the aquarium." It makes perfect sense as I'm saying it, but not at all a moment later. I can't keep my eyes open. My friends have dealt with traffic, parking, taken time out of their day, and have come all this way to see me, but all I can do is drift in and out during their visit. Later, after they've left, I am only aware that they'd even been here because I happen to see a note on the bedside table, scribbled on a paper towel, from Justine: "We'll come and see you at home when you get sprung from this joint."

I get up from my chair slowly, clutching my bandaged chest, and move to the bed. I ache all over. My chest hurts. Breathing is a colossal effort. *This must be why no one wants to be a patient. No one wants to be here! It sucks on this side of the bedrails.* Nurses especially, prefer the other side of things. Can you blame us? On that side, you're the boss, you call the shots. You get to decide when the patient gets the meds, when they get up or go back to bed.

But it's not just the hospital that takes over – illness does, too.

Ray is my nurse tonight. He popped in at the start of his shift to say hey and is back again now. "How're you doing, sweetheart?" He takes my blood pressure and temperature, then straightens out my bed. He gives me a med cup of pills and I don't even ask what they are – or care. I swallow them down. "How was your day?" he asks.

"I moved from the bed to the chair, from the chair to the bed. I walked around the nursing station."

"That's fantastic!" He pats my arm. "After the pain meds kick in, I'll be back to take you on nice stroll down the hall to the atrium. Here you go, sweetie." He places the pills in one hand, a cup of water in the other, and dashes off.

There's a reason nurses wear running shoes.

Later, Ray comes back, gets me up, guides me past the nursing station and down the hallway. It's a long walk but worth it. The reward is the atrium, a huge-dimensioned room, generous with air, light, and space, plus plants and comfortable chairs. Civilization! Why can't more of the hospital be like this, bright, spacious, clean, and inspiring? Along the walls are floor-to-ceiling windows that look out onto bustling University Avenue, known as "Hospital Row," with tall, imposing medical centres lining either side. There's majestic Queen's Park with the provincial government buildings at one end and the University of Toronto buildings – some heritage and traditional, others modern and futuristic – then foreign consulates and embassies, their colourful flags waving in the breeze, lining both sides of the boulevard.

Hey, world, you're still out there. I'd forgotten all about you.

I've seen the wonderment on patients' faces when I've set them up in a chair at the window for the first time after being in bed for any length of time. They look out at the world again, rediscovering it in amazement. That's probably the look on my face, too.

Back in my room, Ray admires the baskets and vases of flowers friends have sent. There's even a bouquet made of fresh fruit — pineapple, cantaloupe, and strawberries, cut into shapes of daisies and roses. He tidies my room and makes me comfortable in bed, tucking me in for a rest. Is it bedtime already? Not yet.

"Is Melissa off tonight?" I ask.

"She called in sick."

Nurse Ray has blond hair, a beautiful smile, nice muscles, and lots of tattoos on his arms. I worked with a nurse who had a tattoo of a twelve-lead ECG on his bicep. "Is it yours?" I asked him. "Of course. It's so I'll always have my own my baseline ECG wherever I go."

We nurses are nothing if not practical.

Later in the evening, Robyn arrives, bursting with her natural beauty and good health. She hugs me and I am embarrassed because I smell. She walks me down the corridors, slowing her quick steps to match mine. She handles me cautiously like I'm a fragile object. In the atrium we sit on a smooth leather couch, and, as promised, she begins to fill in my "lost time."

"Do you remember me and Ivan being there? In the ICU?"

"No, not at all."

"Well, we were. It took so long for you to wake up and they were worried about you. You've always described your ICU patients as being 'in between.' Now I know what you mean. You told me ahead of time what I'd see in the ICU and how you'd look. It helped me to know that beforehand, but even so . . . seeing it, and you like that . . . it was a shock." She shudders thinking about it.

"Nothing prepares you for that," I say.

She shakes her head in agreement.

"It was probably harder for you than it was for me." A recovered patient once told me she had no memory of the ICU, but her husband did and he was still recovering from the experience. I wonder if Robyn is, too?

"I'll never forget how Maria watched you like a hawk," Robyn continues, clearly needing to tell me every bit as much as I want to hear, all that happened. "She didn't take her eyes off you, except for quick glances at the cardiac monitor, then back at you. I felt like a kindergarten child suddenly plunked down in a science lab. "Eighty-six – eighty-five – eighty-two – the numbers kept going down. *The measurements of your life!* 'Is everything okay?' I kept asking her. She looked concerned. I tried to gauge from her face how serious it was. Watching those machines, I felt how it was possible to embrace technology. Then I went back out to the waiting room to check if Ivan had come back to the hospital. He was there when you came out of surgery, but then went home for a while to be with the kids.

"Did they let you come back in right away?"

"Well, no, I stayed out there for a long time before they said I could come back in. I'd been in so many waiting rooms that day – I counted seven in total! Finally, I couldn't wait anymore so I called on the phone at the desk. 'Can I come in to see Tilda Shalof?' Either the nurse on the other line didn't hear me or something was terribly wrong. There was silence. 'Tilda Shalof, can I see her?' I asked again, now in a panic. 'Oh, I'm sorry, dear. Someone was asking me something,' she said. 'Who do you want to see?' This place was making me paranoid. I was thinking the worst. It's like your surgery was a flight and your plane was delayed. A storm is brewing and you're two hours late.

"Call back in a half-hour, dear,' she tells me. 'Half an hour?' I felt desperate, like I'd swum across the ocean only to be told to turn back and wait for further instructions. I almost cried, but I didn't. It was now long past shift change and the nurses had finished with their report when families are supposed to wait, so I worried that something was not right. 'What's going on?' I wanted to run down the hall and yell, 'What's happening?' 'Why is she still on the ventilator at ten o'clock at night, almost eight hours after her surgery? Why have others who went in at the same time woken up and she hasn't?Oh, I had a million questions, but what I needed was for them to look after you, so my questions had to wait."

She sits at the foot of my bed and tells me all that happened, like a bedtime story.

"Ivan called to see if you'd woken up yet and when I told him you hadn't, there was a long pause. I didn't know if everything was okay, but I reassured him that you were resting. He said he was waiting for the kids to get back home and then he was going to feed them and come back to the hospital."

"Where were the kids?" I ask in sudden alarm. "Why weren't they home?"

"They were home, but your brother and sister-in-law — Tex and Bonnie — had taken them to hockey camp and they were on their way back."

"Oh . . . I see. I forgot about hockey camp."

"So, Ivan asked me to call if you woke up or if I heard anything more. I sat down and stared at the clock. What a serious face it had — maybe they should change that up? — but then I couldn't wait any longer. I called to see if I could come and check on you again. Finally, I was told I could come in. When I came in there was the night nurse, Maria. She was standing with a doctor at the foot of your bed. There were both studying you, staring at you like you were a painting in an art gallery. They were concentrating deeply and looked worried, but when they noticed me they smiled.

"'Is she doing okay?' I kept asking them.

"'Her heart is fine,' they told me.

"'Why is she not waking up?' Maria told me she was keeping you sedated and on the ventilator because of the bleeding. 'Not unusual for a major operation like this,' the doctor said, 'but a worry, nevertheless.' Your blood pressure was very low and they'd already given you one blood transfusion and were giving you a second. I asked myself how worried you would be if you had a patient like this."

"Pretty worried," I said. "I guess I gave you and Ivan a scare . . ." I'm beginning to realize how close I came to dying, that I could easily have died if not for all the people caring for me and especially the unknown blood donors who saved my life.

"Then Maria put the siderail of your bed down and helped me move closer. She told me I could hold your hand. I don't know why, but I was scared to do that. I was careful not to disturb any tubes, and I placed my palm on your hand and held it for a long time. Do you remember me doing that?"

I scan my memory bank, but I'm pretty close to E on the gas tank. "No." I shake my head. "Not at all."

"I'll tell you, Til, throughout this entire ordeal, the possibility that you might die had honestly not entered my thinking. I know you'd thought a lot about it, but I couldn't go there. I had travelled across the country, over mountains, Prairies, and the Great Lakes, to go through this with you, and maybe make it a little easier for Ivan, but I did not come here to witness your death. But as I stood right next to you, my hand resting on yours, which was so pale and still, not moving at all – I suddenly realized that you could die tonight. So, all of a sudden I am thinking about death and reviewing my own life. Do you think our death dates are predetermined? My intuition was telling me that it was not your time to die, Tilda. I found myself breathing in sync with you on the ventilator. I saw that we are not the deciders here. There's something bigger than all of us."

"So, what did you do next?"

"I found a washroom and there was a metal bar by the toilet and a red help button. I felt like pushing it. I looked in the mirror, faked a smile, and then gave in to tears. I splashed cold water on my face because Ivan was going to arrive any minute and I didn't want him to see I'd been crying. Then I went back out to the waiting room and took a seat. I looked around at the decor. There were lots of chairs, navy blue with yellow, green, and beige subdued polka dots – not bright neon colours, but not too cheerful either, just in case. A man and woman sat across from me. When he noticed my red, puffy eyes, he offered me a box of Kleenex. In an East Indian accent, he said, 'Very hard waiting.'"

"'Yes,' I said, holding back tears.

"'We wait for . . .' he said, but his wife hushed him by placing her hand on his knee.

"So, I can tell you, Til, there were forty-two chairs, three fake green plants, two living-room lights, eighteen squares on the rugs . . . Counting things calmed me down."

"Where was Ivan?"

"At about eleven-thirty, I heard the elevator door and I knew it was Ivan. When he saw me, he thanked me so much for being here. I could see how grateful he was. Then we walked arm-in-arm down the long hallway to go in together to see you and ask Maria and the doctor lots of questions. 'Is it harmful for her to be on the ventilator for so long? Why is her blood pressure so low? What are all the iv's for? How many blood transfusions is it safe for her to have? Where was the bleeding coming from? When will she wake up?'

Oh, Tilda, you would have been proud of our good questions. We stood around your bed, me and Ivan, Maria, and a doctor and a respiratory therapist and it didn't matter who had what expertise or which titles. We were all taking care of you, worried about you together. But they didn't have the answers or were just too busy taking care of you to tell us more. Ivan stood there looking at you, just touching your arm lightly. It was such a simple, caring examination of the woman he loves, the mother of his children. I think he was afraid to disturb you. He wanted to be able to tell the kids you'd woken up from the operation, but knew he wouldn't be able to do that.

"'What happens if her blood pressure keeps dropping?' Ivan asked Maria. She said that Dr. David was coming in to decide the next move and that he may have to take you back to the operating room and have a look. Then we asked Maria what we should do and she told us to go home and get some rest. She promised if there was any news, she'd call us. I've heard you say this to patients, so I felt it was okay to leave your side. Ivan agreed, so we left."

I absorb these details, her comforting presence, and the soothing peppermint lotion she's massaging into my feet and legs as she continues the story of my two lost days.

"So, we got into the car, exhausted, trying to sort out what was happening. We were halfway home when Ivan's cellphone rang and it was Maria. She told us that Dr. David was there and he was going to take you back to the operating room to fix the problem. Ivan pulled off to the side of the road and stopped the car to talk to her."

"If he stopped the car he really must have been worried. He's always driving and talking on the phone."

Robyn nods and continues, "We didn't know whether to return to the hospital or go home to the kids, but Maria said she would call us when she had more news, so we headed home, talking about nothing, just random thoughts to keep our minds off things. We were almost there when the phone rang again. It was Harry. He asked Ivan if you were okay."

I'm glad I wasn't there to hear that question or Ivan fumbling for an honest answer.

"He said there were a few problems but that you would probably be all right, but he couldn't give the guarantee that Harry was fishing for. He asked Ivan to buy him an Archie comic. He said it would help him fall asleep."

He hasn't read Archies in years!

"Ivan said he'd try but didn't think he could find one at that time of night. He was so sweet and patient with him. When we got home, Harry was leaning over the staircase banister, waiting for Ivan to come upstairs and lie down with him. Ivan said he'd be there in just a minute. I made myself a cup of tea and Harry a hot chocolate – and Ivan poured himself a whisky."

We have a laugh over that. *So Ivan.*

"I told him to give me a swig so I could brag to you later that I'd needed hard liquor to get me through this night! Then I went upstairs to give Harry the hot chocolate and he was still awake, sitting in his bed, fully dressed, staring at his books, all lined up on his shelves. Funny, it was exactly like you would do, Til. I wonder if something like that is genetic? 'You're just like your mom,' I told him and that pleased him. 'Is Mom okay?' he asked me. 'Everything is fine, but they are watching her closely,' I told him. Earlier, he'd made Ivan promise you would be okay. Finally, he went to bed. The phone rang about two in the morning and Ivan, Bonnie, Tex, and I were all still up. It was Maria calling to say they didn't take you back to surgery after all. Dr. David managed to fix the bleeding and your blood pressure stabilized. Then Ivan got off the phone, let out a sigh, and poured himself another whisky. What a relief! It was like fresh air after a storm. I went to bed, but before I fell asleep, I worried about if you woke up and were frightened, but I knew Maria was with you, so I conked out, knowing I had to be rested for the next day."

I am beginning to connect the dots . . .

My head is clearing. I look over at the wide windowsill. Tall flowers, purple and red, stand upright in a glass vase. Today was hot and sunny and the water level dipped down as these intelligent flowers gulped water. Now, in the evening, they take tiny sips, leaving the water level nearly constant. It's *meniscus*, so maybe I don't have pumphead after all? I need to find that wise balance, that clever self-regulation, for myself.

"Do you remember any of what I'm telling you?" Robyn asks.

"Very little. I felt safe and that I was being cared for. That's about it. Oh, and I remember thinking I understood what was happening, but I realize now I didn't."

"Where were you? That's what I kept wondering," Robyn muses. "I felt you were here, but I couldn't find you, which was strange because even though we live far apart, I've never felt like I can't reach you, but during the surgery and when you were in the ICU, I did. It felt like you could easily slip away while I was out in the waiting room, so I needed to be with you as much as possible."

"Was there anyone else in the waiting room?"

"A mother and her teenaged son and daughter were waiting for news about their father, who was undergoing complicated surgery. The mother smoothed her hands up and down their backs as they sat on either side of her. 'What can we do?' the girl asked her mother. 'Pray,' the mother told them and that's what they did."

Robyn stays a while longer, then tiptoes out, thinking I'm asleep and not wanting to disturb me. She's flying home in the morning, but between us there's no need for hellos, goodbyes, or any formalities, for that matter.

The lights have been dimmed in the hallway. I've dozed off and on all day, but I'm still tired. Nurse Ray left his stethoscope hanging on my IV pole. Slowly, I ease myself up and manage to pull it down. Sitting on the edge of my bed, I place it on my chest and listen to my heart and silently thank God for each *lub-dub*, every *tick-tock*. For the first time in my life, my heart sounds strong and healthy. It sounds like a normal heart. *Wow.*

Up till now, I haven't had many rational thoughts, but one occurs to me now – and as grand and over-the-top as it sounds – it makes perfect sense: if every human being could be cared for so lovingly, if we could ensure that every human being's needs were met so completely – world peace would be possible. How hard could it be? Maybe we could even nurse our planet back to health.

11

TRUSTING STRANGERS

Day four post-op. I'm on the mend, may have even turned a corner, but the morning got off to an unsettling start. I awoke to whispering voices outside my room. "The wrong patient," it sounded like one nurse was saying to another. "He wasn't supposed to get it, but he says he feels better than ever."

Mmm . . . There are harmless errors, I thought to myself, but here's something new: a *beneficial* one.

I tried to get back to sleep but couldn't and I lay there, uneasy. Moments later, I hear them again, now chatting about another nurse's engagement – "The party's now, but the wedding's more than a year away. . . ." which somehow leads to a discussion of Indian cooking. One nurse advises the other to fry onions, garlic, and ginger in ghee and the other politely insists that coconut is the essential ingredient. One of these nurses comes into my room, introduces herself, checks my armband, hangs a bag of antibiotic on my IV pole, and plugs it into the saline line running into my arm.

I look up and examined it. Yup, that's the drug I'm supposed to be getting, the right dose, right time, right route of administration, and right patient — *me* — but it got me thinking . . .

It's a good thing that the nurse identified herself and checked my name band because I haven't met her before and she doesn't know me. It's incredibly easy to mix up patients' names and faces. Once, in the ICU, there were two patients, side by side, a Mr. Scotland and a Mr. London. (This sounds like a joke, but it's true.) *One's the country, the other, the city,* I kept telling myself to keep them straight, but a few times over the day, I caught myself addressing them with the wrong name. Luckily, they didn't care or were too sick to even notice, but I had another patient who did. He was angry, but I couldn't figure out why. He couldn't tell me because he was intubated and too weak to write me a note. "His name is Roger," his wife told me coldly when she came in the afternoon to visit and heard me calling him Richard. I felt terrible and apologized profusely. How upsetting for him! He must have felt I'd been taking care of someone else, maybe even worried I was giving him the other patient's meds.

During this hospital stay, I've been given many tablets, capsules, and IV meds. Despite my woozy haze, I know what they're for, their colours and shapes, possible side-effects, drug interactions, and what I'm supposed to be getting, but what if I didn't?

"These aren't my pills," a patient once said to me, handing them back. I checked and double-checked and indeed they were the correct meds, but she was right to ask me to verify. But what if you don't know what questions to ask, or you feel intimidated, or aren't well enough to ask them? Luckily, a friend of mine was. "Hey, what's that for?" he asked his nurse, stopping her as she was just about to give him an injection. "It's your insulin," she told him. He reminded her that he did not have diabetes, though his roommate in the bed next to him did. "Oops," was all she said. He probably didn't find it as amusing at the time as he did months later, when he recounted it to me with a chuckle.

Computerized doctors' orders and medication dispensing systems will likely reduce errors, but it's going to take more than that to keep patients safe. Some of the other factors that cause errors – stress, fatigue, distractions, interruptions, time constraints – are common features of nurses' work, and let's face it, when it comes to medications, it is nurses administering them to patients. Yet, as a patient, you want – no, need – to trust the people caring for you.

I'll never forget the friendly-fire interrogation I received years ago from Dr. Arnie Aberman, who was the dean of medicine at the University of Toronto and a staff ICU physician at the time. He was known for his exacting standards and his habit of interrogating doctors and nurses – everyone, in fact – to make sure we knew exactly what we were doing in our care of patients. He himself was such a conscientious and caring doctor that he would show up in the ICU, at any time, day or night, weekend or holiday, to see a patient. "I'll always come in," he would say. "If I'm giving testimony in a court of law, I can't just tell the judge how the patient was described to me over the phone. I have to see with my own eyes." He always claimed that was the reason for coming in, but I knew he also did it because he was genuinely concerned and wanted to ensure everything was done properly.

One morning on rounds, he began to grill me about my patient, her diagnosis, medical history, tests she'd undergone, and treatment planned for that day. Then he started in on a line of questioning that felt like a cross-examination, but I knew him well enough not to take it personally. It was an intellectual exercise, meant to teach me something, though at the time, I wasn't sure what.

"What medications is your patient receiving?" he started off.

I told him, along with the doses and the reasons for each one.

"Did you change your patient's abdominal dressing today?"

"Yes, I did it earlier this morning." *I spent over an hour on it, so please don't tell me you want me to take it down again so you can have a look at it,* I thought, but he had something else in mind.

"How do I know that you changed the dressing?"

"Besides the fact that I've just told you and charted it, too? And that I signed and dated the wound care assessment sheet?" But these answers weren't what he was looking for. I tried again. "The wound is healing well with a moderate amount of serous sanguinous drainage but no purulent discharge. There is pink granulation tissue around the circumference and the edges are beginning to approximate."

"Now we're getting somewhere. An eyewitness account." He continued his questioning. "Okay, tell me, what's running in her IV?"

"Normal saline at TKVO – To Keep the Vein Open," I added, in case he wasn't familiar with our nurse lingo, "piggybacked with an antibiotic. Ampicillin."

"How do I know there is ampicillin in that bag?"

"Because I just told you I put it in there." *Where was he going with this?*

"How could someone else know what was in that IV bag?"

"They could read the label I stuck on the bag. 'Ampicillin, one gram.' I dated and signed it, too." *What more was required?*

He looked at me askance, eyebrow cocked. "Do you believe everything you read?"

"We're professionals. We trust one another."

"That's a dangerous habit. If you were on a witness stand, and this was all the evidence you could come up with it wouldn't hold up in court. It would be hearsay."

Thankfully, I've never had to testify in court, but how could we do this work if we didn't rely on one another? Yes, it's true you can't be sure something was done correctly unless you do it yourself, but what about teamwork and trust? Both are essential to do this work. And you need enormous amounts of trust to be a patient. (How stressful to be cared for by people you don't trust!) Yet, a healthy dose of *circumspection* on both sides is needed to keep patients safe. You can have all the computers, patient identification mechanisms, and safety checklists in place, but if don't have true partnership, no one *feels* safe.

Years ago, I worked with a very experienced nurse. She had lived in different countries and had many specialties – obstetrics, pediatrics, orthopedics, and, when I knew her, critical care. Victoria was knowledgeable and capable and I had no reason not to trust her until one day I found a large syringe filled with fentanyl hidden behind the sharps container on her side of the counter. Noting the concentration, I calculated that there was 1,000 mcg of narcotic in that syringe. I was shocked. That amount is given to a patient in divided doses over hours, with close monitoring, during general anesthesia for surgery. In the ICU, we never give more than 25 mcg IV in a push dose, and then only if the patient is intubated and on a ventilator. When I asked her about it she didn't seem at all perturbed by my question, casually saying she'd withdrawn that amount by accident and was planning to put it back in the narcotic cabinet later. We both knew it was impossible to return liquid to the original glass vials that had already been broken open. Then she came up with a different answer. She said she had been planning to inject that large dose of fentanyl into a bag of saline and use it for a continuous infusion for her patient. That was a more plausible explanation, but still, it was a huge red flag. Besides, for me it was too late: I had already gone from trust to mistrust.

I suggested we go to the med room to dispose of the narcotic. She said she would do it herself later, but I insisted we go together to "waste" the medication and I would witness its disposal, a practice we do whenever there is unused narcotic. Thinking back now, I should have notified our manager, but luckily, other nurses had their own concerns, too, and they reported her.

Soon after that incident, she was off on extended sick leave and I heard that Victoria was in the process of becoming Travis and was suffering severe pain following gender-reassignment surgery. That provided a possible explanation if she had been "diverting" medication for her own use, but I never found out for sure if she/he was a drug user.

I am a trusting person. Trust is where I begin, unless I have reason to think otherwise. But it seems like old-fashioned trust is becoming scarce. Over the last few years, with the increase in security measures and the tightening of practices to protect privacy in all areas of society, it feels like there's more of a culture of fear and suspicion than ever, even in the hospital, where trust is needed more than almost anywhere else.

For the nurses, one of the first signs of a loss of trust happened when Corinne, our fearless union rep, political activist, and superb nurse, found what she believed to be a surveillance device installed in the medication room, on the ceiling. "It's a spy cam!" Corinne said, appalled. She went straight to our manager in indignation. The administration said it was an "air quality monitor," but we didn't buy that. Someone else told us it was an "inventory control device," but if so, shouldn't we have been informed that we were being watched? Corinne took matters into her own hands and dismantled the contraption herself, with the rest of us standing by, cheering her on.

That incident happened a number of years ago, and looking back on it now, while I still admire Corinne's daring and initiative, by today's standards our outrage seems outdated. Nowadays, surveillance is everywhere; it's the new normal. We recently learned that "undercover" watchers from Infection Control have been covertly observing staff to evaluate compliance with hand hygiene — of course, justified for quality control purposes, but nonetheless, it took us aback. Cameras are now everywhere, certainly in all public places in the big city from parking lots and banks, to schools and day cares, so why not hospitals, too? Increased "security measures" are supposed to make us safer, but why doesn't it feel that way? In the hospital, there are more rules and policies designed to protect privacy, more transparency and accountability, and full disclosure about "adverse events." There are public forums and town hall meetings; reports about a hospital's performance, full financial disclosure of the hospital's budget, the surgeons' rate of infection or incidences of complications for various procedures, even the annual salaries of the hospital's senior administrators (probably to their chagrin) are easily accessible to all. Yet with all of these measures in place, it feels like the public's trust is at an all-time low.

But when you're a patient what choice do you have but to trust the institution and the people caring for you? You're in their hands — literally. Oh, there's been an attempt to rename patients "clients," perhaps to create an illusion that we're "consumers" making independent and rational health care choices. For hospital nurses, *clients* as a term has never caught on. *Patient* refers to a person you *care* about, a client is someone to be *dealt* with. To nurses, *patient* can be almost a term of endearment because it has the connotation of protection and watching over, of tending to. Admittedly, it also carries the meaning of being subdued and obedient, passive and helpless. However, take it from me, when you're the one in the hospital bed — you're a *patient*!

Why *should* we trust the people taking care of us? Some of us have our own reasons not to. Trust can't be promised, guaranteed, or legislated; you can't be convinced or persuaded to trust, and there are no policies, mission statements, or corporate philosophies that will ensure it. Yet you know when it's there and when it's not. But for trust to be effective, it's got to be mutual and reciprocal. It's a *relationship*.

The ultimate sign of one family's distrust was a bright yellow Frisbee. It was hung in a patient's window by her husband, who was dissatisfied with our nursing care of his wife. His hotel room was across the street and we could see him aiming a telescope on the room identified by the yellow Frisbee, spying on us while we took care of her. We joked that the stuffed dog he left on her bed was probably bugged. When he wasn't there, we talked into its plush fur and said silly things. He didn't trust us and we learned not to trust him. All in all, it wasn't a very therapeutic atmosphere for the patient, his wife. Nor was the time that a family brought in a herbal tea for us to give to their mother. We had no idea what was in the strange-smelling concoction and they weren't able to tell us, so we refused to administer it to her. That didn't stop them from sneaking it into their mother's feeding tube when they thought we weren't looking. All in all, it's better for everyone, but especially the patient, if there is mutual trust.

I try to fall back to sleep to escape my unsettling thoughts, but I can't relax. Worse, to my horror, I get a whiff of my body. I stink. My last bath was that luxurious one two days ago in the ICU. I lie in my unwashed condition, too scared to get up and walk to the shower by myself. My nurse left soap and towels out for me and there's a shower right in my room, just a few steps away. There's no reason why I can't get up. I have been given the green-light with AAT — Activity as Tolerated — on my chart, but with the slightest exertion, I feel short of breath and light-headed. How am I going to get to the shower and wash my body myself? It seems monumental.

Still, I can't sleep. My heart is beating rapidly. Breathing is difficult. I try to sit up but feel sore all over and fall back against the pillow. I've never felt worse.

It makes me think of morning rounds in the ICU when we were discussing a patient whose condition had shown no improvement after surgery. He had been critically ill, septic, and unconscious before surgery and was still now, afterward.

An eager resident pointed out to Dr. Hawryluck, "At least we didn't make him worse."

"No, we didn't make him worse," I remember her saying, then adding dryly, "but we set a much higher standard than that."

Here I am, worse than ever. I'm even considering using the call bell or maybe trying to get up out of bed to hunt down a nurse when one appears at the door, but it's a nurse I haven't had before.

"Here are your pain pills, Tilda" she says cheerfully, "and these are your iron tablets and beta blocker, but first let me take your blood sugar and vital signs."

She knows me, but I don't know her and I can't seem to summon the energy to ask her name. It is so important for nurses to introduce themselves and spend a few minutes to listen to their patients' concerns right from the beginning of a shift. It's absolutely necessary if you want to establish trust.

The nurse tells me that my blood sugar is normal. Next, I hold out my arm for the blood pressure cuff. She starts pumping. She pumps and pumps until she's squeezed me up to over 300 mmHg and holds it there.

"That's too tight!" I snap at her. "You don't have to go so high."

She releases the valve, but for some reason the cuff doesn't deflate. I sit with my arm in a clench. I'm fuming, waiting for her to release it. She doesn't. I can't take it. I rip it off my arm. Nonplussed, she flattens it out and is about to try again, but I stop her.

"There's something wrong with that cuff. It's broken. Try a different one," I tell her, but she resumes pumping up my arm.

Why don't you just forget about it? Oh I know, I know, numbers have to be filled in for my blood pressure. *Just make something up,* I want to tell her. I was tempted to do that, once, when I was a young nurse. I was scared to wake up a patient who was peacefully napping when I came into the room to take his blood pressure. *Let sleeping dogs lie,* I thought. On the other hand, what if his heartbeat is irregular or his blood pressure abnormal? I took a look in his chart. The last reading was 128 over 76. I eyeballed him. He looked fine, but you never know . . . so I woke him up and of course he was annoyed and sure enough, his blood pressure was stable at 134 over 74, perfectly normal. I backed off and skedaddled out of there as quickly as possible.

My nurse pumps up my arm again. The room is hot and I break into a sweat. Then a fuse blows. "That's it!" I yell. "Stop! You don't know what you're doing!"

"Your pressure is 118 over 68. Very good."

Oh, I guess she managed to get it to work.

"Now let's see how you're doing with your breathing exercises," my no-name nurse says, unperturbed by my outburst.

I look at the spirometer on my bedside table. *Too hard to reach it, maybe later.* "Could I have my pain pills, already?" *She's late bringing them to me.*

"I gave them to you already. They're in your hand. Here's a cup of water and here's your spirometer."

Who are you, anyway? Why should I listen to you? You don't have a name and you're wearing the same uniform as the housekeeper who swept my room and the lady who brought me my food tray. How long

have you been a nurse? What are your credentials? I think but keep
quiet, stewing to myself.

"How are you feeling?" she asks, watching me while I do my
breathing exercises.

"Not great," I answer curtly.

She smiles *soooo* sweetly at my sour self. "What you're going
through is normal. Many patients feel like this in the first few days
after cardiac surgery and you went through a hard time, losing so
much blood."

Stop being so nice. I look away. *And why are you treating me like a
baby?*

She wasn't, but I'm acting like one. Adults are not supposed to
need the coddling and cajoling we give to children, but sometimes
you do when you're a patient.

I admired Ashley, a respiratory therapist in the ICU, and her way
of talking to patients. We were taking care of a middle-aged woman
who had chronic obstructive lung disease (COPD) and she was
weaning off the ventilator. We wanted to extubate her, but her condition was iffy and we weren't sure if she would "fly." Ashley
believed she'd have a better chance of success if she'd temporarily
use a Bi-Pap mask to help her transition to an ordinary oxygen face
mask. It would help keep open her alveoli, the parts of the lungs
involved in the gas exchange of oxygen and carbon dioxide. But the
mask is tight and uncomfortable and makes some patients feel
claustrophobic. Ashley explained everything slowly and simply.
She held the patient's hand the whole time, urging her along,
praising every tiny effort. The patient coped with the restrictive
mask successfully. Afterward I complimented Ashley on her bedside manner.

"That's how I talk to patients at my other job at Sick Kids," she
said, referring to the Hospital for Sick Children (another of my

father's pet redundancies — "What other kind of children are in a hospital?"). "If we take the time and explain it to the kiddies, and sit with them every step of the way, we're more likely to get their cooperation."

I take my pills with a sip of juice from a plastic straw. Staring at the straw for a moment, a thought occurs to me. Its opening is fairly close to the circumference of my aortic valve. That's the surgeon's workplace; nursing encompasses all the rest.

"May I have a look at your incision, to check that it's healing well?" Amrita is her name, she tells me when I ask, and apologizes for forgetting to introduce herself. I open my gown for her to change my dressing. She gently removes the surgical tape from my skin and cleans my incision, which is dark red with dried blood, only a few inches long, and appears to be closing well. Amrita gives me a box of bandages, cleaning solution, and tape, everything needed for dressing changes, and suggests that I could do it myself. She's right. *The best care is self-care*, as Nurse Deanna would say. *Amen to that.* Patients come to the hospital to work, not rest. As a patient, your job is to do as much as you can for yourself. The more you do for yourself, the quicker you'll get out of here and the better for everyone, mostly yourself.

Suddenly, the patient in the room next door calls out for Amrita, who is his nurse, too. He's always in his room because he's too unwell to walk and also because he's in isolation for MRSA. Before anyone goes into his room, they must first put on the gloves, mask, and gown. Each time the nurses go in, they're in there more than an hour. The moment they emerge, he calls them to come back in, saying he's uncomfortable and asking to be repositioned.

Sorry, Amrita apologizes, but she can't show me the dressing change now, perhaps later? "You know how it is, don't you?" Yes, I do and it's not pleasant being on the receiving end of it. Nurses are constantly being interrupted or pulled away from helping one person to help someone else who needs us even more. These choices can be fateful. Once when I was working on the floor, I popped in to check on a patient. "Will you stay with me?" he pleaded. "I'll be back in a few minutes," I told him and rushed off. When I returned, a few hours later, he had died. It was his time and it had been expected, so it wasn't an emergency, but I felt so guilty that he didn't get his last simple request and died alone.

Let's hope I don't die on you, I'm tempted to call out to Amrita as she rushes off. *Just kidding!*

Where is my nurse? Where did Amrita go? She's left me here to stew in this heat! For some reason, my room is swelteringly hot. Outside it's summer and in here, there's warm air blasting out of the radiator. I sit, fanning myself. Can't the ward clerk call Central Control and get them to fix the thermostat? It's a remote call centre – probably in Nova Scotia or Karachi – but they can dispatch a local technician. I feel *sooooo* hot and sweaty. *Let me out of here! I want to go home right now, this minute! Oh, but please don't kick me out too soon, before I'm ready.*

I know I'm being unreasonable and well on my way to earning myself the worst diagnosis – "difficult patient." When did I go from easygoing and grateful to demanding and obnoxious? I've always said patients are angry at being sick. They take out their anger on everyone around them, the easiest targets being nurses. Here I am doing the same thing. We have lost control of our lives, are forced to comply with seemingly arbitrary hospital routines, have to request painkillers, and wait to receive our meals when it suits others, not when we want them. I don't think I'd ever realized just how far a hospital takes people from their own lives and comfort zones.

Then I start, once again, just as I did in the early days of this journey, to conjure up the worst possibilities; my mind floods with scary thoughts. By this time "mindfulness meditation" and "being in the moment" have completely flown out the window. *What if I go into cardiac arrest? Will they know to call a code? Do they know what the hell they're doing? They're all so young!* I get up out of bed and go out in the hallway, straight to the crash cart, parked up against a wall behind the nursing station where I'd noticed it earlier. Pacemaker cables present and attached, ample supply of ECG electrodes, epinephrine, atropine syringes; defibrillator paddles, charged to 100 joules. Everything is present and accounted for. *Oh, but I see it was already checked this morning at 0745 hours, by Syesha, RN. Okay. Never mind.*

I return to my room to fret about all the "what ifs."

In the afternoon, I am tired but force myself to attend a cardiac information class where I meet other patients, most of whom have worse problems than mine. One woman in her thirties has a tumour on her heart and has been in hospital for almost a month. You have to be mighty sick these days to stay in hospital that long. She looks in better shape than me, but her problem is serious and she's worried. There is a man in his twenties, tall and blond in a light blue bathrobe, who, unbelievably, had triple bypass surgery for blockages in his coronary arteries. He wants to know when he can drive his car and have sex again.

"What about hunting? When can I shoot my rifle?"

How about never? I scowl at him. *You Bambi killer, you.*

A tanned, well-groomed, plump woman who looks about my age says, "I'll be sixty-eight years old this year. Is it too late for me to change my attitude about being heart healthy, like diet and exercise? Is the damage already done?"

No, of course not, the nurse educator assures her.

An elderly, regal woman wearing makeup and dressed in a silk kimono says, "I'm ninety and I'll be satisfied if I make it to ninety-one. I'm tired of doing housework." After the class she corners me to show me photographs of her grandchildren, but I'm in no mood to ooh and ahh and besides, they're not nearly as adorable as she claims.

Back in my room, a lunch tray waits for me. My blood sugar has normalized, but they still have me on the diabetic diet with artificial sweeteners and low calorie counts. I don't have the energy to complain because the food is terrible and, besides, I'm not the least bit hungry.

Not many ICU patients are well enough to eat, much less enjoy food, but I'll never forget one feisty senior who was. Well into her eighties, up and about, she was impatiently waiting to be transferred out to the floor. Since her bed wasn't ready for her yet, and she'd be staying with us for a few more hours, I ordered her a dinner tray. After taking one look at the soggy green beans, the artificial mashed potatoes, and the lumpy grey mass of stew, she was aghast. "What do they take us for, serving this dog shit?" The food insulted her. "The nerve of them!" she ranted. Then the kicker: "If I eat this slop, it will make me sick."

I agreed. It was *sickening.* I wished I had a bowl of homemade vegetable soup, or something similarly soothing, to offer her. Chinatown was nearby and I thought of running out to get the rice congee that I've learned from Asian friends is their comfort food, especially when recovering from illness. Once, a patient's husband asked me for a bowl of soup for his wife. *No soup for you!* I had to tell him, sorry that I couldn't offer his wife that tiny comfort. There is no longer a proper kitchen in the hospital. All "food" is outsourced and produced in a factory off-site. It is impossible to provide a homemade, wholesome meal in the hospital. Why does it have to be this way? It makes us lose faith in the hospital as a place that promotes healing and wellness.

I've completed two circuits around the ward and on the way back from the third, I check out the arrest cart again. Angiocaths, oral airway, chest tubes, intracardiac needles. There's even an open chest cardiac tray to perform emergency open-heart surgery right at the bedside, if necessary.

As I make my way past the nursing station, I happen to see my chart on the rack. We're moving toward electronic medical records but we're not there yet. There's still a paper trail. Mmm . . . I wonder if they would let me read my chart? There's no one to ask and it's probably not even allowed without a hospital official in attendance. Besides, asking to read my chart might make them think I don't trust them and I do.

For me, it's always been one of the hardest things to care for patients who don't trust. There have been some cases when their mistrust is justified. One patient's son refused to have his mother transferred to a floor where a certain nurse worked.

"That nurse almost killed my mother," he claimed.

I found out that his mother had had a feeding tube that had two ports, one for injecting liquid nutrition and dissolved medications, the other for a small balloon to anchor the tube in place. A nurse had repeatedly used the wrong port, causing the balloon to rupture, allowing liquefied meds to spill out into the abdominal cavity. After a long, painful, and *entirely unnecessary* period of illness, his mother succumbed to sepsis and bowel perforation and died.

When a fatal mistake like that happens, trust is irretrievably lost. However, an equally vexing situation is when there's mistrust and suspicion without any apparent reason, especially in the face of every attempt on the part of the staff to win that trust. That was the case with Trevor Sherman and his wife, Francine.

Trevor had end-stage liver disease from cirrhosis and hepatitis C. He lived for years with these chronic illnesses but eventually developed respiratory problems and kidney failure. Pneumonia brought him back to the hospital and eventually to the ICU, where his condition was rapidly deteriorating.

His wife, Francine, who was a nurse, stayed at his side at all times to supervise her husband's care. For five weeks, she lived in our ICU, only stepping away for a meal, a quick shower, or to use the bathroom. "I need to be here," she told me. "I am as essential to him getting better as the medications." But she openly admitted that her vigilance was also due to her concern that we were not caring for him properly. She tried to cherry-pick which nurses were assigned to Trevor and inquired about each nurse's educational qualifications. She quizzed us on our knowledge and rationale for everything we did. She observed us while we gave medications and changed his dressings, and she frequently found fault with our technique. All the while, she kept notes in a journal and on her laptop.

Of course patients have every right to take notes and there are even some good reasons for doing so, but there are times, especially when relations are already strained, that note-taking makes staff intensely uncomfortable. It feels like the family is gathering evidence for a lawsuit and that puts everyone on edge. At the very least, it can give the impression that they are distrustful and wary of us. One nurse found a notebook a patient's wife had left behind. It was wrong of her to have read it, but she did and told us what was written in it. The notebook contained a list of the "good" nurses and the "bad" ones (by the way, there were some excellent nurses on that bad list), along with insults and racial slurs: "Nurse Constance is a nincompoop." "Ashraf should learn English. Must bring an atlas so he can point out where he's from. Wherever it is – he should go back there!" "Bonita needs to

brush her teeth more often. Stinky breath." We wished we didn't
know what she really thought of us.

But with Francine, no matter what we did, we couldn't enter into
a partnership with her in caring for her husband. She was hell-
bent on seeing us as adversaries. Despite talking with her, offering
explanations and constant reassurance, she ignored what nurses
said and listened only to doctors. Eventually she lost faith in them
too. I saw it happen abruptly the day the team sat her down to tell
her there were no more medical treatments that would benefit
Trevor. All we could offer was supportive care.

Why were we giving up on him? Francine demanded to know.
When were we going to start dialysis to treat his renal failure? What
about trying a more powerful ventilator? she asked and specifically
named the machine she wanted. Weren't there new drugs and different combinations that could be tried? Why wasn't he a candidate for a liver transplant? What about a kidney?

At Francine's insistence, dialysis was started, more meds
administered, and further investigations ordered. Offended by
our gentle questions about his resuscitation status, she wouldn't
allow any discussions about anything other than a "full code" in
the event of a cardiac or respiratory arrest.

"Not everything can be explained," Francine said to me privately
after the family meeting to discuss Trevor's treatment plan. We
were back in his room, the three of us – Francine and I sitting
together beside Trevor's bed, where he lay deeply unresponsive
and on maximum life support. "Doctors don't know everything,"
she said to me and to herself, it seemed. "Haven't you ever cared
for patients you thought weren't going to make it and did?"

It is only after a certain period of time has passed and much consideration has been given that doctors will ever say, "There is no
likelihood of recovery" or "Resuscitation efforts would be futile."

Those grim words are rarely used and only in situations when all options have been exhausted. But yes, in my experience, every time doctors arrived at that difficult and painful conclusion, it came to be. However, I didn't think Francine really wanted my answer, so I didn't offer it. It would only end up in a discussion of statistical probability and I was no match for her logical mind. Instead, I asked her the questions we needed to know the answers to in order for us to provide patient-centred care to her husband.

"Tell me about Trevor. What is important to him? What are his values and beliefs? Are these extreme measures what he would want?"

"Absolutely." She was emphatic. "I know for a fact that he wants every chance to live. We talked about it many times and he said he wanted to go the distance. He's not one to give up when things got tough. He's always said he'll go out fighting."

From what she said, I felt resolved with what we were doing, but the bigger problem I had – we all did – was the toxic atmosphere of hostility between her and the team. Far from partners in caring for Trevor, we had become enemies.

I've heard it said that if you have to go into the hospital, you should make sure you have someone stay with you at all times. There's a widespread belief that you need a "patient advocate" to be your watchdog, on guard and ready to fight for your rights. I've heard nurses themselves say they'd stay around the clock if a family member of theirs had to be hospitalized.

If families wish to stay with the patient because they know that the nurses are overworked, understaffed, and not always able to meet all of the patient's need, and they've come to help with the patient's care, that should be encouraged and enabled. However when families come to oversee, supervise, monitor, challenge, micro-manage, and find fault – that is not helpful to anyone, least of all the patient. It all adds to the siege mentality and culture of fear in hospitals.

On a practical level, the goal we have to set our sights on is to ensure that there are enough nurses who have the resources they need so patients can receive the care they need. A harder, more elusive goal is finding ways to create more trust. In my experience, I have seen far more reason to believe that caregivers are doing the correct thing, and have the right intentions, than otherwise. If family members wish to stay with patients, it is best if they are willing to work with the staff to help care for the patient. True partnership is possible. I have seen it myself many times in the ICU where I work. How else could I have been doing this work as long, or as happily, and in the same place, if I hadn't experienced it myself?

As for our relationship with Francine — it only got worse. She continued to try to direct every aspect of her husband's care. She wasn't like some family members who were misinformed, contributing odd or erroneous bits of information, or putting forth strong opinions about things they knew little about. (Most memorable was the patient who demanded that her dying father receive a "brain transplant," something she claimed to have read about on the Internet.)

Francine was intelligent and well educated and in arguments that were a matter of opinion, we often let hers prevail, as in the case when the infectious disease specialists tweaked Trevor's antibiotics and she disagreed with their plan. In one instance, we followed her wish because it caused no harm to the patient and it made her happy. However, the main area of contention was with regard to sedation and pain medication. Francine insisted that those medications be kept to an absolute minimum.

"You're snowing him," she said accusingly. "The sedation drops his blood pressure and then you have to go up on the Levophed. He won't be awake enough to know I'm here."

This was a situation where we felt like we were treating the
family, not the patient, until we were sharply reminded by Dr.
Neil Lazar, the medical director of our ICU, that our priority is first
and foremost the patient's needs; our goal is always to give *patient*-
centred care. Of course we want to be attentive to families, too,
but the patient must come first. Trevor was clearly in discomfort
from the ventilator, immobility, and many other reasons. He was
restless, pulling at his tubes and IVs, thrashing in bed. Francine
would smooth out his furrowed brow with her fingertips as if to
forcibly erase his discomfort. With this clear clinical evidence of
the patient's discomfort, despite his wife's objections, we continued to administer sedation and pain relief as necessary. "The
patient will not be allowed to suffer unnecessarily," Dr. Lazar told
her unequivocally.

Francine started off every day by drawing back the covers to
examine Trevor's body. She took photographs and made notes on
the various sores on Trevor's body, the areas of swelling, oozing,
bleeding, bruising, and leakage that end-stage liver disease and
multisystem organ failure cause. "You're not turning him enough,"
she often complained. "His skin is breaking down."

Our practice did not change because of her comments. Like
clockwork, we turned him and repositioned his body, every two
to three hours, as we'd been doing all along, as we did for all
immobilized patients. We rubbed his skin and dressed his
wounds. Every day, Vince, our ICU physiotherapist, put Trevor's
limbs through "range of motion" exercises since he wasn't able to
move them himself.

Francine watched us with a perpetual scowl on her face, cor-
recting us along the way.

On an impulse, I said to her, "I get the feeling you'd prefer to
be the one giving Trevor's care." As soon as I said that, I regretted

it because it sounded disingenuous, as if I was challenging her to
see if she could do a better job, but I didn't mean it that way. I
really wanted to find out if she would like to participate in her
husband's care because, if so, we could make that possible. But
she looked alarmed and immediately backed right off. Maybe she
realized she did need us after all. Perhaps she was just too tired to
argue with me. She looked absolutely exhausted.

If there's one thing I've learned after all these years it's that
caregivers have to take exquisite care of themselves. They can go
all out, full-tilt, running on empty for just so long. It's impossible
to sustain the arduous work of caregiving over the long haul if you
aren't taking excellent care of yourself.

If Francine wanted to do some of Trevor's hands-on care, it
could be arranged. These skills are easy to learn; they aren't rocket
science – though the knowledge and judgment required to do them
properly is. Millions of caregivers are doing these things for family
members in their own homes. There are many positive ways
patients' families can get involved. Take Mrs. Delgado, instance,
whose husband, Carlos, was in the ICU on a ventilator for almost a
year. She wanted to be involved in his care, so we taught her to
bathe him in bed, care for his skin, shave him, change his sheets,
and suction his mouth. She caught on quickly and it pleased her to
do these things.

"I love this man," Mrs. Delgado said to me as she was combing
his hair one day. Nothing about his intimate care bothered her.

"Don't think we're going to share our salary with you," a nurse
teased her.

Francine loved her husband every bit as much, but she couldn't
bring herself to touch his deteriorating body. She showed her love
by directing his care and by being his protector, but since she
couldn't shield him from his illness, she tried to protect him from

us. What she didn't realize was in order to be his saviour she didn't have to make us into villains.

"You're doing a good job," she said to me one day, suddenly con- ciliatory. "Well, the best you can . . . you see, I've had bad experi- ences. You are a good nurse, Tilda, and there are some other good ones, like Anthea, Kwai, Danielle, and Erin — they are wonderful nurses — but then there are *others* . . ." She gave a shudder. "I won't name names."

I've always advised young nurses not to take what patients say personally. *It's not about you.* Families want to retain control or they need someone to blame and it's often the nurse. They take out their anger and frustrations on nurses or doctors. They blame the hospital or the health care system for what's really bothering them — the fact that they're loved one is sick and has to be in the hospital at all.

I was not offended by Francine's criticisms, nor affected by her corrections, nor bothered by her close scrutiny, but what I did find frustrating and stressful was doing everything in my power to win her trust and making no headway whatsoever. She had made up her mind not to work with us and nothing would convince her otherwise.

"We are all trying so hard to care for Trevor and with you ques- tioning everything we do, watching us every minute, and constantly finding fault, it makes it difficult . . ." I said.

"But I am the expert on him." She pointed at her husband. "I know what's best. He belongs to me."

She had a point. "This is true," I demurred.

As much as anyone belongs to anyone.

We do tend to take over, wresting control away from families. We find it difficult to do our work when patients challenge us or question our decisions, even though they have every right to do so.

We say we want partnership and family involvement, but we keep it strictly on our terms, by our rules. You can sit and watch. You may visit when we say so, but look, don't touch – and don't stay too long! Our authoritarian attitude is born out of concerns for liability, safety, and a long-held belief that we're the experts. But these days, patients are so well informed about their bodies, their health, and medical science, including all the latest research and what tests and treatments are available, that in some situations, it's debatable who knows best. More and more, patients want to be involved. Ideally, it would be as allies and partners, not as opponents or competitors, which is sometimes the case.

"I love him," Francine said, then admitted, "I know I'm a control freak, but it's how I cope. I need to know every detail and I need to see it with my own eyes."

Perhaps this is what Dr. Aberman meant that day when he was questioning me about my patient. You need to see it to believe it. If you don't do it yourself, how do you know it's been done correctly? But, I would answer him now that as ephemeral and unmeasurable as it is, "good faith," on all sides, is also required.

Francine continued to explain herself to me. "If I don't make sure that everything is being done, I won't be able to live with myself afterward. I need to have resolution."

In a family meeting held that day, it was suggested by one of the staff physicians toFrancine that it was time to revisit the plan in place should Trevor go into cardiac arrest. At that point he was still a "full code." He explained to her that in the event of a cardiac cardiac arrest, resuscitation efforts would not be successful, but still, she would not agree to a "Do Not Resuscitate" order. One bold nurse spoke up in the meeting and spelled out for her exactly what a "full code" actually entailed – and didn't spare her the brutal details. Step by step she described the pounding on the chest required and its potential for accidentally cracking ribs, the electrical shocks applied to try to jolt the heart back into a rhythm, and the powerful medications given. The physicians reiterated the impossibility of success in Trevor's case.

"You're all ganging up on me, trying to frighten me. These are scare tactics. You're bullying me!" Francine was fierce and looked horrified. She was furious at us for giving her this bad news.

Despite this frank and honest presentation of the facts, Francine believed otherwise and insisted her husband remain a full code.

"Is this what Trevor would want?" the staff physician asked her.

"There is absolutely no doubt in my mind," she answered.

And so we continued.

Meanwhile, the nursing staff was grumbling. The younger nurses felt intimidated, some ending their shifts in tears and hurt feelings at Francine's undermining of them. A number of the older ones were outraged at being bossed around and felt affronted by her criticisms. It was the main topic of conversation in the staff lounge.

"She should know better. She's a nurse herself," someone said and we all agreed with that.

"If it were my husband, I'd be busy sucking up to his nurses, not making it more difficult for them," someone else commented.

"Funny how she thinks threats and intimidations will get her better care, but it only makes us try to avoid her. Why doesn't she realize that if she works with us, it's better for him?"

The doctors saw how hard it was for the nurses.

"I don't get it," one medical resident said. "Who gives nurses a hard time? Don't people realize their loved one's life is in your hands?"

"In England we would never go this far," a visiting critical care fellow said. "We don't offer treatments that have no benefit. What a waste of money! It astounds me that here, you let families call the shots – they're too emotional and don't know enough about medicine to make these decisions. Maybe the reason you do it is because it's for free?"

No, not free, but sometimes it feels that way. Cost never comes up in these discussions, at least not at the bedside, as it pertains to an individual patient's treatment. I have never witnessed bedside rationing in the ICU where I work. So, why *do* we go to such lengths to continue to offer treatments that we believe are of no benefit to patients? I think we do it because we hate to dash a family's hope, however misguided. We do it in the pursuit of attaining consensus and trust. We do it in an attempt to bridge the gap between the family's beliefs and the doctors' prognosis, which often is at odds. Most of all, it is an expression of our dedication to "patient-centred" care. And yes, there may also be times when it is done to avoid confrontation – even litigation – from a contentious family member.

For nurses, it is not an option to be a "conscientious objector" and refuse to care for a patient because the situation makes you uncomfortable or you disagree with their choices. Even so, some nurses put up considerable resistance, even calling in ahead of time before the start of their shift to plead not to be assigned to her – "I mean, to him" – they corrected themselves. The truth was that we spent much more time caring for Francine, helping her manage her anxiety, providing her with reassurance, explanations, and emotional support, than we did caring for her husband.

By now Trevor was deeply unconscious and every organ in his body was shutting down. Even with dialysis, his fluid volumes, electrolytes, and acid-base balance could not be normalized. His body was bloated beyond recognition and oozing all over with horrible-smelling fluid. His skin was breaking down and in some areas had turned black.

I felt differently than the others. I called in ahead of time to specifically ask to be assigned to their care. *This is the patient I need.* Don't think I'm such an angel: I did it because of something I heard at a funeral years ago. In his eulogy, the rabbi said that the deceased was someone who had devoted herself to her family and community. "She was a woman who had conquered herself so that she could serve others." From that moment on, my own personal "mission statement" became clear to me — to achieve that degree of self-mastery so that I could become the nurse I aspired to be. I've had my work cut out for me and I'm not there yet. So, I continue to seek challenges like this in the hopes of becoming a better nurse, which is also my way of becoming a better person.

I was Trevor and Francine's nurse for two more twelve-hour shifts and got to know her very well and him, through her. Early one morning, a mere three days after that last family meeting to discuss Trevor's code status, I walked in to find Francine sitting beside Trevor's bed, reading a book about miracles. She seemed pleased to see me and to know I would be his nurse that day. "I'm not religious," she said, as if excusing or apologizing for such an unscientific book, "but I am spiritual."

People often say this — I say it myself. For me it's come to mean that I am open to trying various self-help strategies and borrowing wisdom from a smorgasbord of religions and philosophies while consciously avoiding what's difficult or inconvenient, like ritual, practice, and prayer — the *clap-trappings,* as Janet comically calls them. I'm an eclectic "all-theist." But I think Francine meant simply that she believed in a Higher Power but didn't belong to a particular faith.

"I can't let him go," she added, which was the truest thing of all.

Later that day, when the end was near, Francine shifted into higher gear, shouting orders at me and all the others who came to the room to help when they heard the commotion.

"Speed up the drips!" she shrieked.

There were ten IV pumps delivering powerful medications at high rates.

"Nine-nine-nine it!" she shouted, using our private jargon to describe how we max out IV drugs on our pumps that fall 1 cc short of delivering 1,000 cc per hour.

Despite these measures, Trevor's blood pressure and heart rate continued to fall.

"Give albumin!" Francine said, referring to liquid plasma protein that draws fluid that has seeped into swollen tissues back into the circulation and in some situations may temporarily improve a patient's low blood pressure. So, at her request, we did order a unit of albumin and gave it, knowing it would not lengthen Trevor's life, nor add a bit of comfort or dignity, but in the hopes that it might give a dose of peace to Francine.

I doubted it. I didn't believe Francine would ever have peace.

When Trevor's heart went asystolic – "flatline" – and we did not do any further attempts to resuscitate him, Francine seemed to unhappily accept this.

Despite her testy personality and all that we went through together, I became fond of Francine. But, as in most cases, there was no reason to stay in touch after she packed up her husband's things and left the ICU where she had spent so much time with us over those few but long and gruelling weeks. Our relationship had ended, as it usually does with our patients once they go out the door, one way or another.

What brings peace? I often wonder. For me going through my surgery, I had to first know exactly what I'm up against, all the risks, yet choose to fight the good fight, and then let go, surrender to the outcome. As for trust, it has always been my natural state and where I like to stay. When I stray or falter, I do everything I can to find a way back to trust. I have to trust.

Maybe what has to happen is this: patients have to be more trusting and we caregivers have to do more to be worthy of that trust.

In the afternoon, I play hooky from another cardiac education class even though I know I should learn about lifestyle changes, a healthier diet, and daily exercise. I've come to the realization that if I don't change my ways, I am headed for the dreaded "metabolic syndrome" – a precursor to diabetes, coronary artery disease, stroke, and cancer.

Finally I take a shower, all by myself. Pretty pleased with my accomplishment, I take another stroll around the nursing station and stop to chat.

"Look at you!" the nurses exclaim. "You clean up nice."

Then we hear it: "Code Blue . . . Code Blue." Everyone at the nursing station tenses up and leans forward, listening for the location within the hospital. Was the crisis happening on one of the medical wards, or in the food court near the burger joint, or possibly out in the parking lot? I retreated to my room.

Lying on my bed, I pondered the pageantry of Code Blues. There are many actors, each carrying out specific roles, all following a script that varies only slightly. There's lots of behind-the scenes action, high-stakes drama, but in the hospital, where people are already very sick, only occasionally, a happy ending.[*] It starts with whoever is on the scene first, usually a nurse, recognizing that a

---

[*] Instituting cardiopulmonary resuscitation (CPR) or using an automated electronic defibrillator (AED) out in the community have much higher rates of success. Everyone should know how to do these things.

patient is in distress and calls for help. If there is no pulse, the nurse jumps up on the bed to start chest compressions. Help comes quickly and the room fills with people.

The "code" may start out chaotically but soon settles down as the players take up their roles and everyone becomes quiet and focused. (Once, when I was working in the ICU, there was a Code Blue cardiac arrest taking place in a room right next door to me, happening so quietly I didn't know about it.) A doctor is designated as the leader and everyone comes together under his or her direction, egos usually kept in check. When the person performing cardiac compressions gets tired, someone comes forward and takes over. The respiratory therapist manages the patient's airway. After making certain that the compressions are generating an actual pulse, and on direction from the leader of the code, a doctor or a nurse pushes emergency drugs such as atropine, epinephrine, adrenalin, lidocaine, vasopressin, calcium chloride, glucose, sodium bicarbonate into an IV in a large vein in the neck or groin. Someone draws arterial blood gases, runs them to the analyzer machine, then rushes back and reads the results out loud to everyone in the room. From those numbers, we know if the patient is receiving enough oxygen, if the acid-base balance is within normal limits – and much more. If the decision is made to shock the heart, to try to get it back into normal sinus rhythm, the defibrillator is charged up. Pads are put on the patient's chest so the electricity won't burn the skin. "Stand back. All clear!" the doctor says.

(We take great caution with this step, especially those of us who were present the day a third-year medical resident got a shock – literally. His lab coat pockets were overstuffed with loose change, a stethoscope, cellphone, and spiral-bound handbooks, causing it to be so heavy it dragged down and made contact with the metal bed frame. He gave the patient and himself an electric shock. He slumped to the floor and was whisked away to be resuscitated while we stayed in the room and continued the "code." He made it, but unfortunately the patient didn't.)

A "code" can go on for many minutes, even an hour. When it's successful – what satisfaction and jubilation we all feel! When it is unsuccessful and is finally called off, there is a sudden and unsettling calm. The time of death is pronounced. Everyone strips off their vinyl gloves and turns away from the exposed, worked-upon corpse. One by one, they walk away from the messy room, strewn with empty syringes and assorted debris, and return to doing whatever they were doing before they dropped everything and ran in to try to save a person's life. Everyone leaves – except the nurses. We stay behind with the body, wash it, sponge blood out of the hair, and do all the things that nurses do to bestow dignity upon the body of someone's loved one. We tidy the room, dim the lights as if to soften the blow, then go out to bring the family in, offering our arms for support and our words for comfort.

But tonight I'm not on duty. I can relax and not concern myself with all the matters an ICU nurse has to consider upon hearing "Code Blue": Is a bed available in the ICU if the patient survives the arrest? If not, is there a stable patient who could be transferred to the floor? Is there a nurse for the patient? Is a room clean and equipped? Where is the family? Are they at home and need to be informed ever so gently over the phone that their loved one is in a crisis and may not make it? Or are they in a waiting room somewhere, frantic and distraught, needing someone to throw them a lifeline of hope? Since I'm not a nurse right now, I have the luxury of thinking only what an ordinary person would think: *I hope that poor soul makes it.*

12

NURSES EATING CAKE, DRINKING COFFEE

Saturday night. Everyone is either out on the town with friends, having a good time, or else at home, sipping wine and snuggling in for the night. No one wants to be here in the hospital – not the nurses or doctors – or us patients, either.

Shift change. It's 1915 hours and the night nurses, peppy and fresh, rush in to relieve the droopy and spent ones who are moving slower, tallying up fluid balances, and finishing their charting by writing the words – a tad prematurely – that will release them from the responsibilities they've shouldered for the past twelve hours: *Report given to night RN.*

Those going and those coming take up places around the nursing station, ready to give and receive report.

It's still unbearably hot in my room so I'm sitting in my blue hospital gown, in the hallway, on a chair that I've dragged out here. Positioned near the nursing station, I can eavesdrop, watch the action, and vicariously enjoy the familiar activity and aura of intimacy of shift change. I'm smack-dab in between my two worlds.

The nursing station is the usual setup. There's a long table in the centre, counters around the perimeter lined with phones and computers, and, at the back, a rack of charts in dark green plastic binders. (We are still in the process of weaning ourselves off paper.) I listen in on the amusing banter going on at our "water cooler."

". . . I'm switching over to nights, but my body is not happy about it."

"Tell me about it. When I'm on nights, I have no social life."

". . . spent the day cleaning the house . . . my three sons, a husband, and a father-in-law, but not one person in my household who can pee in the toilet."

How I love this chatter! In my ICU, I work with hundreds of people. I know them all by name, am on friendly terms with most, close friends with many, and Facebook friends with quite a few. Recently, a patient asked to "friend" me. Would it be crossing a line to be on Facebook with a patient? It feels that way to me. I couldn't be friends – neither Facebook nor the flesh-and-blood type – with anyone who is currently my patient. The Internet is shaking up old notions of privacy; there's a lot more sharing going on, but some boundaries are still necessary, especially in the hospital. (By the way, on the hospital computers we can't do any social networking, but it's not for lack of trying. There's an impenetrable firewall.)

There's always a commotion at change of shift, and I know one nurse who prepares herself for what's ahead by finding a quiet spot and meditating. She says it helps her get centred before diving into the unknown fray. My friend Mary, in North Carolina, passes a church as she drives to work. "I say a blessing and ask God if He could do rounds with me again this shift, and give me an extra dose of wisdom and patience," she told me once. Then there's the rest of us, who merely plunge right in, hoping for the best.

Soon, the nurses settle down to the business of giving report. Don't worry – we patients aren't left on our own – they are a few steps and a call bell away. They've gone into a tight huddle so I take my chair and return to my room to give them space to exchange confidential information about patients.

There's an art to giving "good report." There's a lot of important – often crucial – information and instructions that must be conveyed in the midst of noise, distractions, and interruptions. You have to be focused and organized in your presentation of your patients' history, plan of care, and remember to mention any pressing work you've left undone that needs immediate attention. You can't just relay facts: a good report also conveys interpretations, opinions, and impressions but manages to avoid biasing or swaying the oncoming nurse. You try to sneak in a helpful hint of how the previous shift was for you and what sort of scene the oncoming nurse is facing. A few "heads-ups" are always welcome! Receiving a good report is the best way to start your shift.

Unavoidably, individual styles come out in our report-giving. I once knew a nurse with amazing panache. She used handover to showcase her own accomplishments as much as the patient's progress. Phaedra's reports were perfect – thorough, to the point, and delivered concisely. "I weaned him off the Levophed and got the blood pressure stabilized. I improved his creatinine, normalized his lactate, treated his potassium, and brought the hemoglobin up to eighty-five from seventy after transfusing two units of blood." She beamed with pride, taking full credit for any and all improvements in her patient, as if she was a one-woman show. Phaedra was a superb nurse – and made sure you knew it!

One of the most memorable reports I ever gave was about a patient whom I'll call Violet. It was a very sad situation. Violet lived a hardscrabble life on the streets of downtown Toronto, working as a prostitute and in the drug underworld. In addition to mental illness, Violet had cardiac damage as a result of cocaine abuse, respiratory issues, and acute kidney disease requiring dialysis. She also suffered a side-effect from one of the drugs she was on. It caused poor circulation to her extremities and her fingers became necrotic – blackened and shrivelled. They were hanging on by mere threads of mummified skin. (Think *Tales of the Crypt*.) That was one of many shocking details that had to be included in my report. In order to give a complete and accurate picture to the oncoming nurse, I also had to describe Violet's bizarre behaviour, like her attempts to rip into her rectal drainage bag to eat her feces; the multiple genital piercings that necessitated delicate perineal care; Violet's unusual "relationship" to a stuffed Winnie-the-Pooh she placed between her legs and "made love to" (there's a more accurate word but this book is rated PG). I tried to keep my composure as I hurried through my report, then rushed away to escape the sheer gnarliness of it all. I was desperate to get home and into a hot shower.

But in the car on the way, I suddenly realized I had forgotten to inform the oncoming nurse about the loose fingers. *What if she came across one of those desiccated, dangling digits – a flying phalange that had come dislodged among the bedsheets?* She'd get a fright and be scarred for life. I pulled over to call the hospital.

"Don't worry. Of course you told me about the fingers," the nurse reassured me.

As I mentioned, a good report prepares you for what's ahead.

The nurses are interrupted from handover by the patient in the room next to mine. He has started moaning, "Take me home, man,"

"Help me, sir," and "Help me, ma'am," over and over. The nurses
haven't finished their reports, but one of them gets up and goes to
his room, first putting on a gown, gloves, and a mask because he's
still in isolation. Another nurse goes to help her. Then, about a
half-hour later, when they come out and as they are finishing
washing their hands, a family member approaches and asks them
to please go back in because the man is still not comfortable. The
nurses glance at each other, yet show no sign of impatience, and
gown up again and go back in.

"Do you want the radio?" I hear one of them ask twenty minutes
later, as she's about to leave again. No answer. "AM or FM?" Muffled
response. "AM or FM?" she repeats. It's not long before they're all
laughing with the instant familiarity of old, easy friends.

His nurse is my nurse, too, and after a reassuring squirt of anti-
bacterial hand sanitizer, she comes into my room, introduces herself as Yolanda, and takes my vital signs. In her crisp, white uniform
she stands out from the rest in their pastel or patterned ones. You
don't see many people wearing white uniforms these days, but it's a
sure sign of a nurse. As she takes my temperature, I see on the lan-
yard around her neck that holds her name tag and hospital ID, the
phrase "I ♥ Jesus." Many patients find that comforting. I do, too.

Good times! It's someone's birthday and cake and coffee are being
served at the nursing station. A green bedspread is the tablecloth
and wooden tongue depressors, forks. Nurses are the designated
celebrators, party planners, and potluck dinner/baby shower
organizers — and the ones who stay afterward to clean up the mess.

Raucous peels of laughter. How rebellious it feels to be cheerful around here! It's not seemly for a nurse to be eating, resting,
chatting, or laughing. Sometimes it's even uncomfortable to tell
patients or family that I'm taking a break. It surprises them, maybe

because nurses are expected to be constantly available, there to meet others' needs, not have any of their own.

(It's always best not to take too long on a break. A nurse once told me that she'd been gone for more than an hour and during that time, her patient got married. She missed the wedding ceremony, but luckily they saved her a slice of cake!)

"They're busy doing nothing," I've heard visitors complain when they see nurses sitting around the nursing station, joking around or in high spirits. I see how it seems that way, but if only they knew how necessary it is for nurses to regroup, think, study, collaborate, socialize, and commune with one another. These things usually take place in off-hours or stolen moments in equipment rooms, hallways, or waiting for elevators. However, the need to debrief and de-stress can be every bit as urgent for nurses as it is for combat soldiers, firefighters, and police officers.

How can nurses offer comfort when they don't feel it themselves? We go to great lengths to keep our feelings hidden from patients, to not let on if we're worried, scared, or quietly freaking out. Then, afterward, we escape – usually off-stage – and let loose. We all know stories of nurses who "lost it" on the job or later, after-hours. Most hospitals make psychological counselling available to employees dealing with job-related – or otherwise – stress.

Sometimes pent-up emotions get the better of us and we need a reminder to rein it in. In fact, we have a discreet sign, a plastic flower that we hang outside a patient's door at times when there is a particularly sensitive situation, like a crisis or a grieving family. It's a visual alert to everyone to show more decorum.

At night, we tend to loosen even more. Laura always used to say she behaved better on days, only swearing on nights. One thing is for sure. Whatever petty conflicts or grievances we have on days, we usually manage to put them aside on nights. We try to come together and help each other. Night shift is hard and it never feels normal or natural to work all night, but what's the answer? Nursing presents unique challenges to staying healthy.

But some of our harmless shenanigans don't help our image. Once, I was sitting in the staff lounge with colleagues, eating cake someone had brought in celebration of something or other. Suddenly, we noticed family members peeking in at us through the window in the door. Nurses aren't supposed to be enjoying themselves. "Nurses just want to have fun!" was our anthem, but "Let them eat cake!" the onlookers must have thought.

In another cake-related debacle, we were gathered and just about to partake of a birthday cake in the "fishbowl" behind the nursing station. Stephanie went off to the pantry in search of a knife, but all she could find was a rather large cleaver, more suited to pumpkin-carving. On her way back, still holding it, she heard an alarm going off in a patient's room. Seeing that the patient's nurse was busy with another patient, Stephanie stopped to remedy the problem. "I hope you're not going to use that on me," the patient said in terror at seeing a knife-wielding nurse at his bedside!

In another weapon-related incident, none of us will forget the stir Nurse Gina created the day she called over the loudspeaker, "Who has the gun? Whoever has the gun, please bring it to the nursing station immediately!" She was referring to an instrument used to staple chest tubes to the suction apparatus, which we called the "gun." You can see how that could create alarm, but it was also pretty funny, too.

FYI to the public at large: if your nurses are noisy or having too much fun and it bothers you, speak up and say so. Know that all you have to do is say, "Please help" or "I need you" and we'll drop our forks, knives, or "weapons" to come to your aid.

—

It's 2130 hours. A nurse is writing in a chart, the telephone cradled next to her ear, reading a bedtime story to her child over the phone. "I'll be there in the morning, sweetie, before Daddy takes you to day care," she says before hanging up.

Another nurse sits beside her, text-messaging her boyfriend.

Beside a bank of cardiac monitors a telemetry nurse oversees thirty-six patients' heart rhythms. An alarm goes off, she looks up, studies the screen for a moment before deeming it a "normal abnormality" (there are such things), and silences the alarm.

I listen to a nurse on the phone speaking to a family member. "I'm just calling to put your mind at ease," she is saying. "I knew you would sleep better if you talked with me before you go to bed. Feel free to call whenever you like and I'll let you know how he's doing. It's our job to worry, not yours."

You have to be extra cautious on the phone. Once, I gave information to a patient's husband and later learned the couple was separated. He was only calling to make sure she was still alive so he could continue to collect her pension cheques. Another time, while talking on the phone to one patient's daughter, all of a sudden I clued into the fact that the background echo I was hearing meant I was on a speaker phone. I had just broadcasted personal information about my patient to unknown people who were also present in the room. Privacy is not only getting tricky to define, it's getting harder and harder to guarantee.

The night is moving along. I hum a few bars from "Strangers in the Night" — *shooby-dooby-doo* — an old Frank Sinatra song. These pain meds are great! Feelin' groovy! *Whoa-oa-oa! I feel good, I knew that I would, now . . . sugar and spice . . .* Thank you, James Brown! Here in the cardiac ward, most of us are getting better — like me: I'm going home tomorrow.

It seems like the nurses are running the show around here.

Haven't seen any doctors tonight, but there must be at least two because I heard one nurse ask another which doctor wrote an order for her patient because she needed to clarify something about it. She asked, "Was it the resident with the blue hair or the one with the purple tattoo?"

(I swear, I don't make this stuff up.)

The din has died down. The hallway lights are lowered. Beddy-bye time for us patients, but the nurses' night is just getting underway. Janet, of Bagel Club renown, pops in for a visit. "Just making my rounds, checking on my babies, and thought I'd see you, too, Tillie." But the wave of heat in my room hits her too and we don't stay in there for long.

"It's freakin' hot in here." Janet fans herself with her clipboard of papers, notes on her patients. "Stick a fork in me – I'm done. Let's get out of here."

We walk to the visitors' lounge and she slows down her brisk steps to match mine.

Janet gives me a once-over. "Jeepers, you're looking a heck of a lot better," she says. "You were in rough shape down in the ICU. Not a healthy-looking specimen at all."

"Were you there?" I have no recollection of visitors.

"You don't remember, do you? We were all there and saw you, stewed, blued, and tattooed. It figures you'd hemorrhage – nurses are always the ones to get complications."

Satisfied with my progress, Janet turns to her *real* patients. "Did you hear that Code Blue yesterday? She was my patient. I'd been following her all day. Vital signs were normal and I didn't have specific concerns – just a bad feeling. I talked to one of the vascular surgeons about her, a guy who was an intern on a floor I worked on many moons ago. Back then, he wouldn't even talk to me, but now that I'm an ICU nurse, he does – go figure. He's one of those jerks

who's always complaining about nurses, how useless and incompe-
tent they are or how many times he got woken up at night, etcetera,
etcetera. 'Go easy on them,' I told him. They're young and have no
one else to call. Anyhoo, I told him I was worried about this patient.
He said, 'What's the problem? She's doing fine,' but I had a bad
feeling about her. Sure enough . . ."

"What made you think something was wrong?" Janet's observations are never vague or ambiguous, but her ability to recognize subtle
clues – some would call it intuition but it's much more than that – is
unerring, absolutely *bankable*. This quality is priceless in a nurse.

"I couldn't put my finger on it, but she did not look right. No
sir-ee, Bob! The operation went well. Her numbers were hunky-
dory. On paper, she was a rose, but in person, not so much. I gave
her iv fluids and took some blood work, but then I had to check out
the lay of the land in the rest of the hospital. Meanwhile, other fish
were being fried and I didn't get back to her until five in the afternoon when she was right on the edge."

"So what did you do?"

"I always ask myself, How can I fix or improve the situation? I
have to do something and I'd rather do it before a patient arrests.
She was chugging along at over forty resps per minute, her heart
rate was one hundred and thirty. I drew an arterial blood sample
and it was absolute garbage – dark cherry red. The respiratory
therapist put her on 100 per cent oxygen. She was pre-arrest and I
needed help, so I called a Code Blue. I wished I could have prevented it, but in this case, I couldn't."

"How is she now?"

"I just visited her in the icu. She's hanging in there. The family
was grateful I made things move along faster. 'You told us to trust
you and we did. We took you at your word. You were the only one
who saw there was something going wrong.' They appreciated that

I hadn't walked away. On the floor, some nurses are reluctant to engage. We're not used to that in the ICU. If we see a problem, we have to do *something*. We don't walk away. 'You saved her life,' the family said. Isn't it the best feeling in the world?"

We sit on the couch for a while, thinking about this, the best feeling in the world, until it's time for Janet to walk me back to my room and for her to get back to work.

A man in a dark green uniform carrying a toolbox arrives at my door. He's here to fix the heater in my room. We chat briefly and I hear his Farsi accent. "What did you do back in Iran?"

"Mechanical engineer," he said with a wry grin. "No work here."

It's a reminder of other people's concerns and the world outside of the hospital — something I'd completely forgotten about — and countries where many people have a lot more to worry about than the temperature of their rooms. Sheepishly, I thank him for fixing my problem.

A pizza delivery guy has arrived. The nurses have ordered in food. Believe me, you don't want a hungry nurse! There's a nurse I know who brings a bag of celery for lunch and drinks coffee all day. How much energy does that provide? Would you want her caring for you? On the other hand, one hungry nurse went down to the food court late at night, just before it closed, to buy a Subway sandwich. She returned in a state of shock, visibly shaken.

"What happened?" we gasped when we saw her, rushing over to her with a chair.

"I was buying a sub and suddenly I hear weird sounds from the back of the dining area, you know, where the Coke machine is? I went over to check it out and there was this guy moaning, his pants down around his ankles, jerking himself off. Where's a security guard when you need one?"

She was still carrying the plastic bag with her submarine sandwich, so I couldn't resist:

"Was it a six inch or a twelve?"

How we howled with laughter!

Yes, such juvenile jokes and sophomoric pranks help to get us
through the night. Call it nurse bonding. Sometimes our work
makes us as needy as our patients. There's the heavy-duty labour
that results in neck, back, and muscle injuries – as much as con-
struction workers – and the hazards of night shift. Sometimes even
more draining is the emotional labour. All in all, it's a risky career
we've chosen and hospitals aren't usually very healthy environments
for nurses. We have to work extra hard to stay healthy, but I know
many who don't.

"We're parents, nurturers, caregivers," Janet was saying one
evening in the staff room. "Between home and work, we're holding down two jobs and not taking care of ourselves because we're
too busy taking care of everyone else, patients, their families, and
our own families, too."

She would know, I thought, because she does all of those things.

"Yeah, tell me about it, girlfriend," chimed in Nina. "They say,
'God can't be everywhere, so he created mothers.' I say mothers
can't be everyone so that's why there are nurses. We give, give, give,
but it's never enough."

Nina would know, too, because she was none of those things.
She was one of those nurses who always feels hard done by. We all
have moments like that, but she never seemed to rise above it as
most of us do. That night Nina was particularly bitter in the wake
of a heated encounter with her patient's wife.

"Her husband isn't getting better, so what does she do? Blame
the nurse! I feel burned. I gave so much and next thing I know, she
reports to our manager, saying that I had crossed the line, that I was

'unprofessional,' too emotional. I swear I'll never get involved with families again."

Ah, being professional — contained, businesslike, definite of your boundaries. If only expertise, skill, and knowledge were all that was required, it would still be a tall order. On top of that we're also supposed to be mindreaders, purveyors of cheer, hope, comfort, kindness, and inspiration. Most of us start out idealistic and enthusiastic, trying hard to provide all these qualities to our patients, but many of us fall short at times along the way. There's so much in a hospital that can break your spirit.

There's one aspect about being "professional" that's still a challenge for me. It's the distance you're expected to keep, that stance of formality that is required. I've always treasured the more human moments when I've ditched the "professional stance" and allowed myself to be real, when I've chatted one on one with patients and their families, joked around, shared a laugh or something of myself. Boundaries can be hard to establish because of the intimate, familiar quality of nurses' interactions with patients. For example, at the end of that unintended group conversation with the roomful of people on the speaker phone, just before hanging up, the daughter said, "Give Dad a kiss from all of us." Would they say that to any other "professional"? I admire nurses who use their individual flair, personality, and humour in their interactions with patients. They put their very selves into their toolbox. I love what my friend Rosemary once said, "When I go into my patient's room, they get *me*. I'm the treatment."

It's good to be real and human, but in balance. Some people can't see beyond initial impressions. We don't always do a great job of managing our image. I learned this lesson long ago, on one of my first shifts as a new graduate. I was working with Hannah, an excellent nurse whom I looked up to as a role model. At one point, she checked her watch and said, "C'mon, let's go. It's time to flip the steaks." I was offended by her crude, off-the-cuff words, so callous and at odds with her otherwise professional demeanour, but then I figured, so what? Did it matter if Hannah was a bit rough around the edges? She was kind to patients and clearly knew the importance of repositioning immobilized patients to reduce the incidence of pressure sores. Who cared if she talked like this, nurse to nurse? It didn't change my opinion of her and I've long since learned to see beyond the brash talk or seemingly "unprofessional" behaviour of some wonderful nurses.

Being professional – that's the easy part – but patients expect so much more! In addition to all of the above expectations, at various times we're supposed to play the roles of mother/father, brother/sister, enforcer, confident, teacher, friend, coach, and mentor – not to mention ordinary angels and everyday heroes. Unlike most patients, my expectations of my nurses are more modest. With all they have to deal with, if they give me the correct meds and stay alert to problems, I'm satisfied. Most patients want their nurses to make them feel safe and comforted. Some even want a relationship. They like it when their nurses show emotions, but only if they are in synch with what they are feeling; nurses who don't show their emotions are deemed hard-hearted and cold. Can you imagine a profession where emotional expression is a job requirement? Welcome to nursing.

But I'll admit, at times we can be too *real, too human.* Oh, I've seen some inappropriate things in my day. A nurse who wore outlandish earrings that dangled to her shoulders. Another nurse with a habit of resting his feet up on the desk at the nursing station in full view of the public. One time, I saw a nurse chowing down on a *full-course* dinner – chicken wings, French fries, corn on the cob while sitting right outside her patient's door. The family was gathered around the critically ill patient's bed, and the nurse was contentedly eating her dinner in front of them. She was either oblivious to their crisis or at least wasn't going to let it ruin her appetite.

Then there are inadvertent *faux pas* and bloopers, like the nurse who was leaning on the dialysis machine when her long hair got caught in the wheels. It sounds painful, but her extensions snapped right off and she wasn't the least bit hurt, though her braids gummed up the circuit and brought the machine to a standstill. She was laughing so hysterically — along with her patient — she could barely call for help.

Nurses aren't the only ones who blunder. Once, a staff doctor arrived for a family meeting. He sat down with the distraught family and proceeded to tell them bad news. The complicated operation he'd just performed on their mother had been unsuccessful and her condition was very grave. I watched the family's expression move from shocked to puzzled to bemused and relieved. I realized what was wrong. I tapped the surgeon on the shoulder and informed him he was talking to the wrong family. Wow, that was an awkward moment.

Then there was a small, silly mishap that still makes me chuckle. During rounds one day, a staff hematologist was speaking to the team, outlining a patient's rocky course of chemotherapy protocols. For some reason, he happened to look down at his leg. I watched him slowly peel off a sock from his pants, stuck there from dryer static. He merely stuffed it into his white lab coat pocket and continued on without missing a beat. I admired his aplomb.

I've had my own cringe-worthy moments. Not the worst indiscretion, but one of the most embarrassing happened years ago when I was still working with Laura's Line. An enthusiastic foodie, and onto a new health kick, I had bought a jar of Loblaw's Savoury Seven-Bean soup and ate it for lunch. Delicious and nutritious, full

of fibre and especially *beans,* later that afternoon, I began to experience its explosive *side-effects.* I had to beg various nurses to cover
for me as I kept madly dashing out to the bathroom, each time
trying to make it to a different location, so as not to be identified
with the trail of stink bombs. It didn't take long for Justine to "sniff"
me out. "It's you who's going around here spreading the love!" she
said in her booming voice. Busted! "This one you can't blame on
your patient." Yes, we had been known to occasionally blame our
own gaseous emissions on our innocent, unsuspecting patients.

I tiptoe out of my room and look down the long, deserted hallway.
Not a soul around. I feel like I'm playing hooky – but remind myself,
I'm a patient; I'm off-duty.

How short the night seems at home in your bed sleeping and how
long it drags in the hospital when you're working! There've been
times when I've had to remind myself to keep the faith, that the
night would eventually come to an end. There have been moments,
though, of such intense fatigue that I managed to muster only the
minimal wakefulness required to do my job safely, and not a drop
more. Often I recall a quote by F. Scott Fitzgerald that I like: "In the
real dark night of the soul it is always three o'clock in the morning."
Sure enough, even now, I look at my watch. It's ten to three. Once,
in the middle of a long night shift, I asked Maureen, a hardworking,
seemingly tireless nurse, "What do you do when you feel tired?"
I sat down out of my own fatigue to hear her response. "I don't allow
myself to think about myself," she answered still in motion, in the
midst of mixing a medication for her patient. "I just keep going."

For me it's more of a challenge to stay so focused, especially at
night when I'm tired. Sometimes my imagination can get carried
away, and I'm not the only nurse who's like this. One night in the
ICU, I stood at the window in my patient's room, staring out at the

downtown deserted streets, the traffic lights changing needlessly, unused parking lots, and empty, lit-up skyscrapers. *A crime could easily be committed,* I thought. *There would be no witnesses and the corpse won't be found until morning.* I felt someone creeping up behind me. There was a breath at the back of my neck. A whisper blew into my ear and a velvet voice purred, "Perfect conditions for a murder, don't you think?" I twirled around to see Valerie, a nurse who wrote true crime stories in her spare time. "Wouldn't those icicles make the perfect murder weapon?" She pointed out long, sharp ones hanging from the ledge of the floor above. "When they melt – poof! – there goes the evidence. Something to think about, isn't it?" She turned and went back to her patient.

I come out of my room, bleary-eyed, but still can't sleep. The nurses at the nursing station look tired. I wonder if they've taken breaks or had a chance to rest. I hope so. If they do, they will be more alert and safer. Believe me, you don't want a tired nurse giving you your meds or taking your vital signs.

Yolanda sees me and gets up. "Are you having pain?"

No, I feel fine, but I ask if they mind if I sit out here for a while with them.

"Feel like you're missing out on the convo?" another nurse asks.

"Sort of," I admit and then, on an impulse, ask, "Hey, could I read my chart?"

"Go ahead," he says with a nod and hands it to me. Either I've caught them in an unguarded moment or they've allow me access because of my insider status.

I leaf through the pages, reading the story of me, told in point form, graphs, and numbers. Medical history, lab results, medication orders, consults, reports, consent forms, test results, progress notes, even my discharge summary, all ready for me to leave in the morning – it's all here. The handwritten notes of the doctors of various specialties, nurses, respiratory therapists, physios, chaplain, etc., get intermingled, so your eye always gets drawn to the most legible entries, which often belong to nurses. I know one doctor who says he never reads nurses' notes, only doctors'. That's a shame. He'll miss out on important information. On the other hand, I've seen ICU residents write their daily progress summary on their patients based entirely on information cribbed from nurses' notes.

"Progress notes" are a log of events, sometimes organized in "SOAP" format, starting with Subjective data of what the patient says, then Objective observation. Assessment is what is gleaned from your actual examination, and then there's the Plan of care. Every few years, a new charting style is rolled out, along with a team hired to teach and implement it, then evaluate its effectiveness. I've heard that in some places "narrative charting" is coming into vogue. It allows patients to record their experience, to tell their stories in their own words. It reminds me of an Israeli newspaper that for one day invited poets and writers, instead of journalists, to report the news. "The clothes flapping in the breeze, warmed by the sun," conveyed the weather as vividly as a meteorological report.

Reading my chart is an unsettling experience. I kind of wish I hadn't. It's yet another case of TMI – Too Much Information. I saw in black and white that from 1230 hours to 1355 hours my heart was stopped: ischemic time. Then, later, in the ICU, I was restless and delirious. I read the nurses' assessment of my condition, how they washed me, handled my bodily fluids, and cleaned me. It's all here, my overuse of the narcotic pain pump and my extreme anxiety. There's even a note dating back a few years about my cantankerous behaviour in the ER: "Hostile, demanding to be seen immediately." *How embarrassing!* As for reading your own chart? I wouldn't recommend it. What good can come of it? And it feels like I've intruded on the staff's territory, infringed on their rights. Caregivers deserve privacy, too, from us. We should let them do their work in peace.

It didn't take me long to read through my fairly thin chart, but some patients have charts so extensive they are piled high in tall stacked volumes. Once, I had a patient who had a droopy eyelid and I mentioned it on rounds. To the team, it seemed like a new and ominous finding, possibly indicating a neurological problem. An MRI was ordered, along with other tests. Later, ploughing through the voluminous chart, I read that twelve years ago, the patient had brain surgery for a seizure disorder, leaving her with a weak eyelid. Upshot was, the MRI was cancelled and we returned to focusing on the patient's current problem.

Peoples' health histories can be so complex and charts are invaluable records, but the challenges to organize all that material, get it online, have it easily accessible to all the professionals caring for the patient and yet protect patient privacy is a huge and complex undertaking; a single, comprehensive, integrated electronic chart still eludes us, but we're well on our way and I'm sure it will happen one day soon. Until it does, it's also up to us to be responsible for our own information, keep track of records, tests, results, reports, lists of medications, and so on as best as we can. Maybe in the future our record will be so accessible and interactive that we could monitor our medical conditions and take on even more responsibility for our own health care.

But while the move to electronic charting and computerized medication dispensing machines are improvements, they have changed the way we work. For example, to chart a patient's vital signs, I have to physically leave the patient altogether or merely look away, log on, go through screens, and enter the data. Likewise, to retrieve a medication, someone has to cover my patient so that I can leave the bedside to go to the medication station, log on to the computer, flip through a few screens to open the door of the cupboard or refrigerator to select each drug I need. Back in the days of yore, our nurse manager used dollar-store tin muffin trays that had a cup for diuretics, sedation, inotropes, antiarrythmics, and so on. Medications were kept at patients' bedsides, with narcotics the only drugs under lock and key. In some ways, life was simpler back then. Though I do remember one time, I arrived home from work, reached for my house key, and discovered it was the narcotics key. I had to go all the way back to the hospital to return it. That wouldn't happen anymore. Now there are no keys to worry about with the high-tech security measures in place. We access medications with our individual "biometric profiles." A scan of our fingerprints opens the locked door. Only time will tell if these measure will improve patient safety.

Computerized charting will reduce transcription errors and eliminate illegible writing. It will also help protect patient privacy so I probably won't have the experience I had recently when I was standing in a crowded elevator next to a cardiologist who was flipping through a patient's chart. I could easily read the name, address, diagnosis, and the treatment. With an electronic chart, it's not as possible for health care workers to trespass into friends or celebrities' electronic charts, which are more secure than paper ones. There are undoubtedly additional benefits that I can't even imagine, but there's still one thing I have against computers: they take me away from patients. Time and attention spent staring into an inanimate screen when I'd rather be at patients' bedsides, caring for their bodies, undistracted by technological gadgets, fully present, face to face, being with them and listening to their stories.

I sit at the nursing station, still in my hospital gown, and start to feel chilled. Nurse Yolanda drapes a warmed-up blanket around my shoulders and places a cup of chamomile tea beside me. How does she know I feel chilled?

She guides me back to my room and gives me two pain pills.

"Is this normal?" I ask her about my darkening incision.

"Yes. Red, purple, then back to your natural colour. That's how a scar heals."

On her brown skin, too? I wonder, but feel too shy to ask. I chuckle to myself, remembering a Nurses' Week celebration where there were raffle prizes to be won. A Jamaican friend who forgot to bring her glasses and asked me to read it to her.

"Golf clubs . . ." was the first item on the list.

"Don't want it," she said.

"Day at the spa . . ."

"I'd love it!"

"A visit to a tanning salon . . ."

"Don't need it!" she said, both of us sharing a dry laugh at that.

I look at Nurse Yolanda. I know nothing about her other than she loves Jesus and is a good nurse. We didn't get to know each other, but lots of times it's like that between patients and nurses. A relationship isn't always necessary for a therapeutic encounter to take place, but I do crave some connection to the people caring for me. I can't stand to be strangers for long.

Yolanda guides me to my bed. I made it myself this afternoon. It took me a long time and I didn't do a great job. When patients complain that their bed linens weren't changed, it's a reliable indication they are capable of doing it themselves. *The best care is self-care.* We patients have to do as much as we can to help ourselves get better. Maybe there are even ways we can help the people caring for us to do their work.

"Why don't you pull a mattress in here, for a nap?" I ask Yolanda. I've certainly done it on night shifts, but she looks aghast at my suggestion. Taking a rest, when it's been safe to do so and when trusted colleagues were available to spell me off, has helped me get through many a long night.

Ahh . . . I sink down. "Sleep, nature's soft nurse." A line from Shakespeare floats into mind, out of the blue. These drugs are making me wax poetic. I close my eyes and see tiny bursts of red, purple, and white fireworks behind my lids. Whatever they've got me hopped up on, keep it coming. It's a lovely trip.

I settle back and wait for sleep to come. . . .

But I can't sleep. I'm too excited to go home and see my kids who thankfully, as I requested, have not visited me in here – or at least I don't remember them being here.

"Sleep, God's free medicine," Kate, a nurse friend, says. Maybe that's what patients need the most – a good night's sleep – and to be kept amused while nature cures the disease, to paraphrase the old French philosopher Voltaire. Maybe I'll go out there and ask Nurse Yolanda for something to knock me out, but oh, how I hate it when my patients make me into their drug dealer!

13

BABY STEPS

Ivan has gone off to hunt down a wheelchair. I wish him luck. This is a hospital — he'll never find one here! I wait for him outside my room, sitting and grinning, triumphant at my accomplishment. I made it. Open-heart surgery on Monday and home on Sunday — six days — pretty good!

Nurse Yolanda came to say goodbye to me at the end of her shift this morning. "You were a good patient." She paused to think it over. "Yes, a very good patient." I think she meant I didn't have many complications and wasn't too demanding.

A cardiology resident checked me out and has pronounced me good to go. My blood sugar has normalized, vital signs stable, incision healing well. My hemoglobin is still low, but that will take time to improve. There's a list of meds I'm on — a beta blocker, aspirin, iron supplements, and painkillers — and a nurse offers to explain them all to me. No worries, I tell her, I know this stuff inside out. I'm chomping at the bit to get out of here! Okay, she says and gives me a large handbook of information for the cardiac patient, highlighting its main points. No lifting more than ten pounds for six weeks. (The weight of a watermelon.) Showering is okay but there is no bathing until the incision is healed. No driving for six weeks. No sex until you're able to easily walk up and down a flight of stairs. (Is that because the bedroom is up there?) If you have questions or concerns, call us anytime, night or day.

Eventually, Ivan shows up with a wheelchair – he's nothing if not tenacious – and I pile into it my vases of flowers and bags of gifts and then walk beside it, leaning on it for support as I move toward the elevator. *I'm busting out of here!* A hospital is no place for healthy people. I walk through the front revolving door without a care in the world. My only debt is one of gratitude and a new sense of obligation to take better care of my health. The hospital's only request of me is to complete an evaluation form about my hospital stay because they aim to improve patient satisfaction. They want to know about my "patient experience," like how long I waited for tests and procedures, whether staff was courteous, and if my expectations were met. I have no criticisms. It's like my father's old joke about a perfect wedding – "The bride was too pretty."

It's a glorious morning! I stare out the window at the world that's still there, waiting for me to be a part of it again. The hospital world envelopes you so completely that the real one outside vanishes in your mind.

We stop to pick up a few groceries at the supermarket. Ivan tells me to wait in the car, but I follow in after him. I need to test-drive my new heart – not new exactly, but it feels that way. I wouldn't miss this exciting field trip for anything! On the shelf, a bottle of ketchup! Pickles! It's still summer so there are baskets of sweet plums and juicy peaches! *It's a whole new life for me.* Yogurt! Cherries! Cornflakes! Olives – yes!

"You're not supposed to lift anything." Ivan rushes to take the cereal box from my hands. He's hovering, like when we drove home with our newborn baby.

When we pull into the driveway, the kids run out to greet me. Harry unloads the car and Max throws his arms around me, wrapping me in a squeeze so tight, it makes me gasp.

I may pass out.

"Breathe, Mom," he tells me.

"You're part pig now, Mom," Harry says. "How cool is that?"

I agree, but as much as I love the pig, it's not exactly a compliment. He must realize this because he hastens to add, "The pig is a very smart animal, Mom. It suits you."

Max wants to see my scar and looks at it in fascination. He likes those crime investigation TV shows, so maybe I look like a stabbing victim to him?

Everyone is so happy to have me home – even Phoebe the cat comes over to purr and weave in between my legs.

First thing, I take a shower to wash off all residue of the hospital. I dry myself off and, in my own bathrobe, pad into my office to greet my books. *It was touch and go there for a while,* I tell them, *but here I am. I made it.* Maybe there are a few too many of you. It's time to give some away. It suddenly strikes me as an odd activity to hold on to *things.* Right now, possessions don't mean as much as before, but I'm sure in time, I'll get back into the joys of shopping.

I look over the instruction pamphlet the nurse gave me, but I can't remember what she said. Why did they put me on a beta blocker? How long do I have to take iron? Why am I taking aspirin and what dose and for how long? For pain, they've prescribed oxycodone (a.k.a. OxyContin, the trade name) and it says take two tablets, every four to six hours as needed. Should I take them now or only when I have pain? My nurse tried to explain all of this to me, but I didn't listen, too eager to leave. Now I'm too impatient to read the instructions, but Ivan helps me sort it out.

I'm exhausted from not sleeping, from pain, the blood loss (my hemoglobin is seventy, almost half of what I came into hospital with), and from the sheer relief that it's over. I crash on the new maroon leather recliner I find in our family room. Ivan bought it as a surprise; a must-have for every convalescent!

A tap on my shoulder. Ivan peers down at me sunk into the depths of the recliner. Hours must have passed. "Let's go for a walk. Once around the block."

"Later," I promise. "I'm too tired."

"They told you how important it is to walk. C'mon, let's go."

"Let's not and say we did." I drag myself upright and slowly trudge along the sidewalk, just behind him, each step a supreme effort. I make it only a few steps down the street and am ready to turn back. I can't go farther. I look one hundred years old and feel ancient.

"You'll do more tomorrow. It will get better," he says. "Each day, you'll get stronger. You'll see."

For the next two days, Ivan doesn't leave my side, attending to my every need. But the third day he has to get back to the office and he's worried about leaving me alone. Friends will be visiting throughout the day, but he's hesitant to go. "I'll be back in a few hours," he tells me, placing the cellphone, TV remote control, pain pills, and a glass of water beside me.

"I'll be fine," I tell him and of course I am.

As soon as he gets home, he starts to grill me. "Did you take your pills? What did you eat today? How far did you walk?"

He's a nag. For dinner he fries iron-rich steaks and slimy liver to boost my iron, but I can't eat a thing—certainly not that. He yells at me for not doing enough and at other times for doing too much, like when he catches me unloading the dishwasher, slowly, stopping, out of breath.

"You still haven't learned to be a patient, have you?" He takes a stack of dinner plates out of my hands.

"What does it require?"

"Patience. You have none, but that's you," he says with a sigh.

"Unfortunately, yes."

"Time for your walk."

I've recovered from the dishwasher, now it's time to move.

"I can't. I'm too weak."

"A few more steps than yesterday," he coaxes me. I follow the leader.

We stop, halfway around the block. "Am I a difficult patient?"

"You're a pain in the ass," he says grimly, "but worth it," he adds, grinning.

Over the next few days, I spend most of my time in the recliner, eyes closed. Not asleep but taking a break from being awake. In the evening, I look forward to the reward of my bed. If I pop a few of those Oxy-babies, I sleep all night, too. I take one and in a few minutes there's a jolt of pure pleasure that melts into a calm, robust, glowing feeling of well-being. *Pain? Who cares!* I'm not looking forward to stopping them. How easy it would be to become dependent on them; I have to be careful. It could happen without even knowing it.

Each morning, at the exact same time, the phone rings. It's the hospital's automatic check-in system. "We care about you!" it starts off in a standard-issue, electronically generated voice. It asks questions about my incision, pain, constipation, activity, and mood. I punch the # key for yes and the * for no to answer each question. "We care about you," the voice repeats before clicking off. Right. Some house call.

Ivan, on the hand, is a real nurse. He oversees my diet, gives me my pills, and makes sure my incision is healing. He monitors my pain, energy, and exercise. I read an article about "cardiac spouses" that says they "often feel overburdened and that their needs are forgotten." They haven't met Ivan. He's a nurturer through and through and is thriving on this new project of taking care of me; he puts his whole heart into it and has never looked happier.

I pop two more pills, not for pain, but to avoid pain and remind myself that OxyContin is a highly addictive neurotic – I mean, *narcotic.* I could get $50 on the street for one of my tablets of "hillbilly heroin."

Throughout the day, friends drop by bearing flowers, choco-lates, get-well cards, a tray of lasagna, and pots of soup. Laura and gang have left a bunch of funny movies with a note: "Don't bust a gut!" The ICU team sends me a gift card for Tim Hortons worth $100. That's a lot of coffee, something I usually love and have every day, but now I can't drink coffee, tea, or much of anything. Food tastes strange, slightly off.

Visitors get a shock when they see me as an invalid, weak, and pale, lying there on the recliner, not doing much of anything. They hug me carefully, sensing my fragility. Does seeing me give them an inoculation, like a tiny exposure that confers immunity? Do they get a tiny guilty pleasure knowing it's not them? I have felt both ways, at times, about patients. It's hard being on the receiving end of sympathy and concern.

"How *are* you?" some say gently, as if the question itself might be too much for me.

"You must be so glad it's over," one friend says, more conversationally.

"I'm glad I made it." I'm operating on that level, still amazed at having survived. It's an unexpected gift of gratitude but also a new responsibility to bear.

I'm happy when visitors come, then after a few minutes I want them to go. *Thanks for coming, now please leave.* They can't win with me. I try to be gracious but usually doze off during their visit. It's strange for me to have visitors and not be able to jump up to greet them or make them a cup of tea or a meal. Ivan takes care of that as well as being the gatekeeper, making sure I don't overexert myself, kicking out visitors who stay too long.

As soon as they leave, it's time for a painkiller.

The next day, the electronic "nurse" calls again. Maybe if I hang up an actual person will call and we will have a real conversation. But I guess there once was a time when telephone talk seemed unnatural, too. It puts me in mind of one of my worries about my profession: what is happening to face-to-face, hands-on nursing care? It's beginning to seem like a rare and precious commodity. I'm sure it's acceptable for marketers, radiologists, writers, editors, architects, salespeople, and programmers to toil in the "electronic workshop," but if your work requires building, making, doing, communicating, observing, feeling, being present, emoting, empathizing, witnessing, or listening – all essential nursing activities – a live human presence in real time is required. I know a public health nurse whose work involves teaching, counselling, and consulting, but she always says with a touch of smug pride, "I don't touch patients." I guess she means she's strictly a "knowledge worker," which is how nursing is branded these days by the universities where nursing is taught. Lots of research, policies, theories, and "new knowledge" are being pro-duced there, but patient care is accorded lesser importance. There's a disproportionate amount of thinking over doing. We now have researchers, scholars, and intellectuals in our profession, but not enough people willing to do the yeoman's work of skilled caregiving – an imbalance that is going to have a huge impact on our aging population – in fact, it already has: there's a worldwide nursing shortage.

And why is moving away from the bedside always seen as career advancement? It puts me in mind of Margaret, who was a fabulous hospital assistant. She helped the nurses with patient care in a professional and compassionate way but was thrilled the day she was offered a "promotion" to a ward clerk position. "Now I can use my brain, not my body," she said with pride. In her new position, she gets to wear her own stylish clothes instead of a uniform, sits at a desk, answers the phone, and works on a computer. Many think that hands-on work is unskilled or brainless. *No one wants to get down and dirty!* Even nurses themselves have been known to say that trained monkeys could do some of the tasks we do. I don't see it that way. To me, nothing about caring for patients is trivial, inconsequential, menial, or routine.

In fact, this point came home to me one day at work when I happened to be riding in an elevator with the hospital's CEO. He wore an elegant tailored suit and I, wrinkled green scrubs and a lab coat with a ketchup stain on the sleeve. (At least I hope it was ketchup.) He makes more than $700,000 a year – and I make, well, considerably less. (For the record, a full-time senior nurse in Ontario makes around $85,000.) I don't begrudge him his lavish salary. He has duties and responsibilities I can't even imagine, along with a skill set that is way beyond me, but neither do I bemoan my very decent income. But think of this – if you're a patient, who're you gonna call? Which of us is of more use to you? In your time of need, who do you want to show up at your bedside? A patient needs a nurse more than a CEO and that's why I'm glad to be one.

Thanks for the virtual house call, but the nursing care I value can't be phoned in.

I've napped all day, but night comes and I'm exhausted.

I sit up in bed. Something is wrong. I feel chilled. Ivan piles blankets on top of me but I can't get warm. My teeth are chattering. I take my temperature: 37.1* Celsius, higher than my usual of 36.0.†

A low-grade fever. My first thought – sepsis! Overwhelming infection! Bacterial endocarditis!

A few minutes later I take my temperature again. It's 37.5.‡ I call the cardiac hotline, which puts me through to the ward where I was a patient.

"Is Melissa on? Ray? What about Yolanda?" "My" nurses, the ones who know me, the ones I knew and trusted are the ones I want.

"They aren't working tonight."

Ahh, the mystery of nurses' schedules. Even Ivan hasn't cracked the code of mine. They're like Sudoku puzzles – endless configurations and combinations.

"Could I speak with a nurse?"

"I'm a nurse. Can I help you?"

"I'm eight days post-op aortic valve replacement and I have a fever. What should I do?"

"How high?"

I've taken it again. "37.6."§ Can she hear the barely contained hysteria in my voice?

"You could take a Tylenol," she suggests with a hardly concealed "d'oh" in hers.

---

*   98.8 °F

†   96.8 °F

‡   99.5 °F

§   99.7 °F

"Good idea." I thank her with an imperceptible note of sarcasm in mine.

But what did I expect? This is the correct response. Stay calm. Think it through. Monitor closely. *Be a nurse.*

"A mild fever is common after surgery," the nurse says. "Keep an eye on it. Call back if there are any further problems or if the fever persists. See how you feel tomorrow."

I knew that.

Horrors! I have become one of those high-maintenance patients who always think the worst, whose anxiety is off the charts. I pop two Tylenols and one painkiller, then another. They get rid of pain and just about everything else, too. Such a sweet trip off to la-la land.

I deserve it, don't I?

Soon, a wave of pleasure spreads through my body. I smile to myself.

Ahh . . . this part I like. I could get used to this.

14

SLOUCH ON THE COUCH

My surgery was in August and I've spent most of September crashed on the recliner. I haven't accomplished much. My email inbox and voicemail are full, untouched. Messages from friends, unanswered. My loving family has been waiting on me hand and foot. I feel stronger every day, my daily walks are getting easier. The only problem is a familiar one but hard to admit. I know exactly what it is.

"I think I may be a little depressed," I say to Ivan.

His exasperation flares. "Tilda, you need to get a grip," he says. "What do you have to be depressed about? The worst is over. It went well."

"I know it makes no sense . . ."

"Have you gone for your walk today?" He looks out the window. For days it's been hot and muggy and now the sky has turned dark and overcast. A late-summer storm looms, about to be unleashed on the city.

"It looks like rain," I say.

"I'm sure it will pass."

The rain? Of course it will.

Sitting in a fire truck . . . I accidentally release the emergency break
. . . crash into cars that explode into flames . . . a bleak Chinese
labour camp . . . I've been imprisoned for crimes unknown and am
forced to turn tricks for a dirty peasant in a smoky opium den who
comes after me in a rage with a knife when I try to escape from his
clutches . . .

Terrifying nightmares linger all morning, like a bad aftertaste.
The beta blocker – along with every other "aol," "ilol," and "olol"
– posts nightmares on "side-effects-may-include" list, yet millions of people use it without a problem. It is highly effective in
controlling the heart rate and strengthening the heart's contrac-
tions and decreasing its workload, but I wonder if it's what's disturbing my sleep.

I spend the day suction-cupped onto the recliner, heavy-lidded
and groggy from the narcotics. Lethargic and lazy like . . . well, a pig
is purported to be. When I wake up three hours later it feels like
three days have passed.

The kids are back in school and the Jewish New Year approaches.
Fall usually feels to me like an exciting beginning – but not this
time. Prone on the recliner, I watch Ivan roasting a brisket, stir-
ring chicken soup, rolling matzah balls, baking a honey cake. Only
my thumb is moving as I channel-surf the TV. Not movies or sit-
coms that require concentration, albeit minimal, only mindless
reality shows about overweight brides who go off to boot camp so
they can squeeze into their too-tight wedding dresses or cat-
collecting hoarders living in misery and squalor.

"Mom, these shows are sad," Max says. "Why are you watching them? Are you a *sad-ist?*" He tries to change the channel, but I snap at him — *just leave it.*

The smallest things irritate me and I lose my temper over nothing.

"Looks like someone got up on the wrong side of the bed," Max says when I scold him for a puddle of spilled milk on the counter. (At least I didn't cry over it.)

Harry and Max arrive home after the first day of grade six and grade nine respectively, noisy and eager to tell me about their day, but I have no patience to listen to tales of an already-lost brand-new pencil case or the strict math teacher, "who gave us homework on the first day of school. Can you believe it, Mom?" Max asks, incredulous. All I could think of is that I only hope they don't notice that when they left for school in the morning, I was on the recliner and this is where they find me again in the afternoon. Phoebe, the cat, has had more exercise today than I have between stalking imaginary mice, grooming herself, and chasing her tail.

I place a sandwich down in front of Max, who attacks it ravenously.

"Don't wolf it down . . . like a . . . wolf," I say in annoyance.

"Mom, you're a writer. Can't you come up with a better simile than that?"

I retreat to the recliner, fuming.

"Looks like someone got up on the wrong side of the oxygen mask," Max says, laughing at his own joke, which, I have to admit, is pretty funny, but I can't even fake a smile or a chuckle.

Harry goes to his room and Max sits down to watch my shows with me but becomes distracted by my incision. He gazes at it, mesmerized, as if he's trying to imagine what lies behind it.

"Don't stare," I say, immediately regretting my impatience.

I accomplished the impossible but now can't handle everyday life. Even the electronic "nurse" gets on my nerves. If I punch in the "correct" answers, she moves on. If not, I am taken down a pathway of increasingly longer menu options. It infuriates me how the personal touch is becoming obsolete. One day robots will be caregivers for us baby boomers. But I have to admit, when friends come over to offer some of that human contact, I'm so irritable they probably wish they'd sent one of those robots instead.

Visitors come bearing good wishes and thoughtful gifts – home-cooked meals, scented soaps, and the latest bestsellers. Joy brings me a plastic multicoloured ball that bounces off crazily in wobbly, unpredictable directions that in my slightly stoned state I find wildly amusing. But when friends ask, "How are you?" in their sincere and solicitous way, I spare them the details. The truth takes too much energy.

"What were your symptoms?" the curious ask. "Was it a bypass? A heart attack? A murmur? I have a murmur, too! Why didn't you tell us sooner?" Some ask too many personal questions or launch into accounts of their own medical woes or those of their cat. The worst is when they give advice. *Don't give me advice!* No one really wants advice, especially unsolicited advice. I'll never forget all the useless advice I received when I was a new mother, especially about breastfeeding. "Feed the baby!" "Don't feed the baby too often!" "You aren't producing enough milk – the baby is hungry!" The cacophony of advice was so loud, it drowned out own my inner voice telling me how to care for my baby. The only thing worse than getting unwanted advice is receiving wrong advice. My friend's mother was having bad headaches. "It's because you wear your hair in a ponytail," her bridge club friends told her. "Stop pulling back your hair so tight." Meanwhile, she had a pituitary tumour.

Luckily, her own intuition that something was wrong brought her to the doctor in time to have it successfully treated.

No advice! No questions! Don't offload onto me your own fears! Don't pay me a visit if it is for you to perform a good deed or to fulfill a sense of obligation. Come if you're not going to flinch or pity me or make it worse or harder for me. Just be with me, sit with me, I tell them and then doze off – or pretend to.

Annie, a close nurse friend, knows how to visit. She makes one of her composed, signature salads with exotic greens, edamame, and toasted sesame seeds. She whips up another favourite with Asiago cheese, balsamic vinegar, apples, and figs. She then sweeps the kitchen floor and organizes my cupboards while I try to eat. Even this gourmet delight, so lovingly prepared just for me, is hard to get down. Nothing tastes delicious. I have lost my appetite for food – and life.

Another friend asks me eagerly if I had a "near-death experience."

"Did you go to the other side? Was there a bright white light?"

No, none of that, I'm sorry to disappoint.

A third friend is angry at me and lets me have it.

"I can't stand the way you dealt with this," she says straight out. "You kept it to yourself. You didn't let anyone help you. I could have organized a car pool for your kids, meals for months. Why did you only tell us all at the last moment?"

"I didn't want to worry you. I could only tell nurses."

"What do they do differently than the rest of us?"

"They knew how to help me in the way I needed. They listen but take a step back. Try it. Imagine you're a nurse."

She pauses. "I get it. I'm listening to hear what you need, not what I think you need."

Exactly.

Later in the afternoon, the doorbell rings, but I don't answer it. I hide out on the recliner. Later, on the doorstep, I find a bag left there by another friend named Janet. Inside it are all the fixings for a Sabbath dinner – a pot of warm soup, *perogen* (a South African Jewish delicacy) and a braided challah. In a little box, there is a sparkly heart threaded on a silver chain.

"We have wonderful friends," Ivan says. "See how everyone cares about you."

I know this but can't feel it. None of these kindnesses make me feel better, as they are all intended to do. I want to be left alone to feel sorry for myself in peace.

In my case, is depression a passing emotion or a medical diagnosis? Is it negative thinking or a real illness? Of course I would acknowledge it in patients, but I can't muster the same respect for the symptoms of depression in myself, especially when, as Ivan logically points out, there is no reason for it.

The next day after Ivan has gone to work, the kids are at school, and I'm sucked into the recliner doing nothing, I suddenly start hearing my heart pounding madly in my chest. I start breathing faster, then faster, to keep up with it. My chest tightens. I have difficulty swallowing. Something is wrong. I call the cardiac hotline.

"My heart is beating," I tell a nurse, any nurse, in a rush.

"That's good. It's reassuring, isn't it?"

"But I hear it beating. It's eighty per minute."

"Help me understand," she says, sounding puzzled. "Do you want to hear it beating or not?"

"I just want to know if it's normal to hear your own heart."

"Of course it is. You're just aware of it. Maybe you're having an anxiety attack?"

"No, it's not that," I say. What a relief. My heart is okay. Maybe it's like the new furnace we put in last winter. It made different

noises, working in an unfamiliar way. Eventually I stopped noti-
cing the sound, only that it kept the house warm.

The next day Phoebe the cat has taken over my spot on the
recliner so I move to the couch, but it's not comfortable – too
upright and hard with rough, sturdy fabric. We chose it for dur-
ability and economy. Who knew I'd need a cocoon to hibernate in,
not a serviceable piece of furniture upon which to sit?

The only company I can bear is the TV. In the morning, it's fashion makeovers that make me dissatisfied with my clothes and want
to trash my entire wardrobe. Home decorators ease me gently
through the long afternoon.

"I love beautifying other people's houses," one designer says,
"but my own is a disaster." He's like me. I readily take care of others
but learning to take care of myself, especially my emotional health,
has been one of the biggest challenges of this whole experience. Self-
care is the best care, but sometimes the hardest to accomplish.

Then, Oprah's exhortations to "keep a gratitude diary" and "be
my best self," which only make me feel even more inadequate,
especially when I watch the example of Monica, a woman who
developed a massive infection after childbirth and had to have her
arms and legs amputated to save her life. Her uppermost thought
was to make it home so that she could be a mother to her kids. "I was
still here," she said. "I can still love my children. I have a loving
husband." Now, that sounds like a woman who has conquered herself so that she could serve others. Normally, I would be inspired
by the example of her courage, but now it only makes me ashamed
for my lack of it.

Similarly, I compare my problem to my patients' battles with
life and death. I try to draw strength from recalling the bravery and
dignity of so many patients I've cared for over the years, but these
comparisons also discourage me. It's completely irrational to be

weepy and tragic about my happy situation, but that's what I feel. It makes no sense.

In the evening, I chase the cat off the recliner and lie back on it to watch more newlyweds squabbling about their out-of-control spending habits and controlling mothers micro-managing their spoiled kids' lives and planning over-the-top bar mitzvahs and sweet-sixteen parties for them. Then it's time for two painkillers and off to bed.

I fall back to sleep and enter straight into a nightmare of being nine months' pregnant with a litter of puppies. The sound of them barking, clamouring inside me is what wakes me up.

I get up and go into the bathroom to step on the scale and I see I've lost ten pounds.

Lose weight the open-heart surgery way! The new diet sensation! Don't try this one at home, folks!

The next morning, when the phone rings at the set time, on an impulse, I decide to short-circuit the system by punching in the "correct" responses to each question, regardless of the real answer, thus officially bringing to an end my relationship with the "e-nurse." *Yay, I won!*

I return to the recliner. I'm supposed to walk, increasing the distance each day, but I'm afraid to leave the house. I want a cup of tea, but it's too much effort to get up and boil the water. The phone rings unanswered. The TV screen goes blank. (The kids have shown me how to fix it, but I can't be bothered.) I bounce the pretty rubber ball Joy gave me and watch it careen off in random directions.

When Ivan gets home from work, he peppers me with questions. "How are you feeling? "How far did you walk?" "What did you eat today?" "What did you do today?"

Bad.

Not far.

Nothing.

What did I do today? I got up from the recliner to get the remote control where I'd put it on the kitchen table so I'd be able to report I'd done something.

Even Phoebe looks at me in reproach, her whiskers twitching.

"Are you having pain?" He holds out the bottle, poised to give me pills.

Yes. Not really. Kinda-sorta. Okay, I'll take a few of those puppies. I had open-heart surgery, didn't I? I could get more of them if I wanted. What doctor wouldn't renew this prescription? But am I on the road to drug addiction, an intervention, then packed off to "celebrity rehab"? I had a neighbour once who had to go into detox to get off these painkillers. It could easily be me, too. I take two more and decide here and now to make these my last. Cold turkey. From now on, it's over-the-counter painkillers only.

"You have to force yourself to do more each day," Ivan says.

"I am trying." I hate the whine of self-pity in my voice and hope he can't hear it.

"It would help if you would be more positive."

"I'm trying to be."

"There's no trying. Just *be* positive. You have so much to be thankful for. Stop feeling sorry for yourself and obsessing about your heart." He stands over me, looking down at me ensconced on the recliner. "There are other things going on in the world. Like your kids, for example."

Or his birthday a few days ago. Oh, by the way, Happy birthday, Ivan.

"You're dragging yourself around like an old lady. You're a young, vibrant woman. Let's go for a walk around the block. You'll feel better."

I'm tired. It takes a lot of energy to feel this bad. I long for my bed. Is it time for bed yet? It's only five-thirty in the afternoon.

"I think I'm depressed," I say, staring off miserably into space.

"Oh no, not this again." Ivan comes to sit beside me. "The problem with you is . . ."

That gets my back up. I brace myself.

". . . that you can't deal with discomfort."

Is that all you've got? "Actually, I have a very high pain tolerance."

"I'm not talking about pain. I said discomfort. You can take pain, you just can't handle being uncomfortable. For you, that's worse than pain."

Yes, and I'm uncomfortable in my body and in my mind. For some reason, I think of the kids at camp. To them, feeling healthy and happy every day is like a right, the natural order of things. When they're faced with even minor physical challenges, they feel affronted. Even as adults, when we get a cold, many of us have such meagre resources to cope. I thought I'd feel great by now, three weeks after surgery. I certainly expected I would feel better than ever after surgery and hadn't anticipated such a long and arduous recovery. *Who knew?* I certainly never thought I'd be thrown into this state of intense and debilitating *discomfort* – a sensation that feels lodged in my soul and weighs down my neck, my forehead, right down to my toes.

I look at Ivan. He doesn't entirely get it – maybe because he's never felt this himself? He is all concern and caring, with a dash of impatience. I feel for him; it can't be easy being around a depressed person. It's, well, *depressing*. Thankfully, it doesn't have that effect on him. Over our years together, he's seen me through many ups and downs – upheavals that had nothing to do with weather, success or failure, work, love, or stress. I hardly understand it myself. Is depression created in the mind by destructive thought patterns?

A personal weakness? A learned behaviour? A genetic inherit-ance, imprinted in my DNA with an identifiable marker? Produced by faulty biochemistry? A spiritual quest? A moral failure? All of the above?

Ivan reminds me of what I have to be grateful for (it's a long list), to be more positive (I will try), and to keep moving, walking every day (I am.).

"Maybe you should see your doctor," he says. It's a comment that surprises me because Ivan doesn't usually give much credence to a problem like mine, a problem that looks like if you only tried harder and exerted more effort and self-discipline, you could shake it off and pull yourself together. If only this was a garden-variety sadness I could talk myself out of, or exert will power over, I would, but I've come to the conclusion that I can't. It's beyond me; this much I now know.

15

CHANGE OF HEART

"The most important thing is for you to get started on a cardiac rehabilitation program," Dr. Drobac says at my six-week checkup. In cardiac rehab classes, he explains, I will learn about a healthy lifestyle, how to reduce cardiac risk factors, and will have the opportunity to start exercising in a monitored, supervised environment.

Bo — rrrrringgg. Pshaw on cardiac rehab! Probably a bunch of old geezers in baggy sweatpants, attached to electrodes, strolling on tread-mills. More preoccupation with my heart. I want to put my heart problem behind me, throw off patienthood, and get back to being normal and *light-hearted* again.

Dr. Drobac recommends a particular program that is for women only. "Women have different needs when it comes to cardiac rehabilitation."

"Like what?"

"For one thing, women have more stress, especially if they work outside the home. They are looking after everyone else and don't always take care of themselves."

You got that right — it describes a lot of women I know.

Together we look at my ECG and echocardiogram results. He admires Dr. David's beautiful handiwork and points out the significant improvements in my heart function. "You have a healthy heart now, Tilda," he says, then sits down to work out some fateful arithmetic.

"Well, let's see, how old are you?" He looks at the year of my birth in my chart. "You're almost fifty, so let's say fifty. You have a tissue valve and let's say you get fifteen years out of it and in all likelihood you will. That takes you to sixty-five, then you can get a new valve and most likely have it inserted minimally invasive, by angiogram." He reminds me about the single-dose blood-thinner tablet in development that simplifies anticoagulation. "It will be available by then and at that time you may opt instead for the mechanical valve, which will give you another twenty years, taking you to eighty-five or ninety. If you keep making healthy choices and take good care of yourself, you could live to a hundred."

I like this hopeful math, but so much can happen. I've never taken anything for granted, much less now. He reminds me about taking antibiotics before dental work to prevent bacterial endocarditis, gives me the go-ahead to drive, discontinues the beta blocker because it is no longer needed (and agrees it may have caused the nightmares), but does want me to continue with the daily two tablets of low-dose aspirin, something he recommends for most women and men in my age group.

"How are you feeling?" He looks at me closely. "Depression is common after cardiac surgery," he says, opening a door I refuse to enter, still clinging to the hope that I can fix myself by myself. As for the cardiac rehab classes, I turn them down, too.

[It's time for another Public Service Announcement: Don't do as I did, folks! A recent study has shown that patients who participate in cardiac rehabilitation cut their risk of death by 50 per cent due to changes in diet, exercise, and lifestyle.]

"What did the doctor say?" Ivan asks when I return to the waiting room.

"That my heart is working well and I should come back in six months."

Ivan thinks this is wonderful news and of course it is, but he expects me to act like my old happy self so I fake it with a big smile. Maybe if I give him the "right" answers, too, like I did with the automated telephone questions, he'll leave me alone. The moment we get home, I am wiped out and head straight for the recliner.

For the next few days I keep company with my chubby brides, pageant-bound tots and their obnoxious stage mothers, and the glamorous L.A. tattoo artist and her bad-ass entourage. Today on *Dr. Phil,* three sisters natter at one another about the distribution of their aunt's will. "It's a choice," Dr. Phil says to them. "You can choose to put energy into feeling bad, into perpetuating all of this anger and negativity. Or you can stop it right now, in this very moment."

Maybe that's my problem. I have to stop the negativity – but how?

As the day wears on, stopping the negativity becomes even harder. I am sitting in my office, staring at my books, when I begin to feel my hearting thumping. It's pounding. I take my pulse. Eighty at rest. *Too high.* Something is wrong. The worst possibilities crowd my mind. I take my pulse again. Eighty-four now. I pick up the phone and call Dr. Morse, who opens up an appointment for me right away.

"It looks – and sounds – like you're having an anxiety attack," she says the minute I walk in but examines me thoroughly to rule out any cardiac problems. We chat briefly and she asks me how I'm feeling, but all I tell her is "fine." Calm and reassuring, she advises me to come back tomorrow, but after seeing her, I feel better. When I get home, I call to cancel the appointment.

"I try to see what the bride sees," says a TV-wedding consultant. "I had a bride who chose a strapless dress with a sweetheart neckline and mermaid skirt and it looked beautiful on her at the first fitting, but now she says, 'It's too much dress. It makes my head look tiny.' She wanted it taken in all over. I didn't agree, but I supported her decision because my job is to see things as she does. I am there to help the bride get what she wants, to help her have her perfect wedding and feel beautiful on her special day."

Now that's what I would call "bride-centred care"! Nurses have the exact same challenge — to see the patient's perspective. Only then can we offer what is needed, not what we think is needed. Problem is, I can't offer that same empathy to myself right now.

I flip to another channel, where a perky self-help guru advises, "Hug yourself. Smile, even when you don't feel like it. Make a list of things that cheer you up."

I try out these things, but they feel artificial and contrived. Even Max senses the ruse. "What's wrong, Mom?" After school he comes over to sit beside me on the couch.

"Nothing," I say, but I can't fool him.

He tries to cajole me, picking up his old riff. "It looks like someone got up on the wrong side of Oprah's couch."

Determined to get a reaction, he tries again. "It looks like someone got up on the wrong side of the bestseller list!"

"Still working on your routine?" I ask with a weary half-smile. "It's funny, sweetheart," I say but can't manage a genuine laugh or smile.

"Tough crowd," he mutters as he goes up to his room.

—

Today I was reminded of the grandiose pledge I made to myself before my surgery to one day work toward better health care for all. But on the radio I heard a patient tell about how having to wait too long for radiation and chemotherapy caused her cancer to spread. She was forced to go to the United States for treatment there and feels the Canadian health care system has let her down. I can't imagine the terror of not being able to get life-saving treatment. I can't bear the thought of people not receiving the health care they need. It has never happened to me or any patient in my care, but the problem of inadequate resources and access to health care is real for some. But too often, the public evaluates the entire health care system on the basis of their singular experience, on how well their own needs were met. When patients say, "This is a good hospital," they mean, they got better here, the doctor had good bedside manner, the nurses were nice, and they didn't have to wait too long to be seen. How can we get beyond caring exclusively about our personal needs and move toward a consideration of what's best for the kind of society we want to live in? Besides, why can't everyone have great health care?

We can fix the problems: improve efficiency, ensure access, contain costs, reduce overcrowding in ERS, and improve wait times. New and expanded roles for nurses and other health care professionals could meet more peoples' needs. More nurses — especially in the community and in people's homes — would reduce costly hospital stays. Nursing isn't the way to solve the problems, but it would go a long way toward a solution. Overall, we have a good thing happening here, but sometimes it feels like I'm the only one who thinks that way.

But even I would have had difficulty navigating the system if I didn't know it as well as I do or didn't have a family doctor to guide me through it. I would not have been able to interpret information and would have been even more anxious about the hospital and the tests I had to undergo. Important details might have been missed. Maybe patients need someone like a wedding consultant to plan their hospital "event" — someone to listen to your concerns, field questions, quell jitters, make referrals, coordinate appointments, keep you on track. Being a patient is a big job to tackle all by yourself.

Thinking about the problems of health care have put me into deeper gloom and doom. Why don't more nurses stand up to protect and speak out for Medicare in this country? Nurses are so close to the reality of peoples' lives and know the effects of poverty and inequity on health. We should be the loudest advocates of all for quality health care for everyone.

I sit, mired in my thoughts, fretting over the health of the health care system. The kids are busy, getting ready for hockey practice.

"What's wrong, Mom?" Max asks, coming over to check on me before they leave.

"I'm worried about the health care system."

He pats my back. "Don't worry, *bubbelah,* the health care system can take care of itself without you for a while."

The next day I go back to see Dr. Morse, who suggests I take an antidepressant.

We all have our own mythologies, the stories we tell ourselves to get through hard times. My story is that I should be strong enough to overcome depression with my own willpower and determination, that relying on drugs is the easy way out. Yet, I have never passed a similar judgment on a patient. I have great sympathy — even affinity — for patients with mental illness. It's just another example of the perplexing dichotomy between how I care for my patients and how I care for myself.

"Why not take meds?" a friend says. "Everyone's on them these days. The stock market is a disaster. There's a financial crisis. It's enough to make anyone depressed."

That reasoning I don't get. Antidepressants are for depression, not life's challenges. For me, the only thing I ever found depressing was depression. Sure, stress and real problems can lead to depression, but that's not my situation. Are medications the only way to way to feel better? All I know is that I can't fix this by myself.

I'm listening to a cryptic telephone message from Janet: "Meet us at the farm. Be there or be square."

What farm? Where? Why a farm, of all places?

"No questions," Janet goes on, anticipating my thoughts. She only gives me directions and the admonishment, "Just show up."

Janet, Jasna, Stephanie, Kate, and Edna are waiting for me, greeting me at the entrance to Pine Farms with its rolling hills, trees in autumn colours, a pick-your-own apple orchard, and a country kitchen serving homemade soups and pies. They present me with a huge bouquet of flowers and I accept it with a deep bow, like I'd just performed a recital at Carnegie Hall. How women excel at making moments special.

"Lots more people wanted to come," says Janet, "but I said no. Too many cooks spoil the brew."

"There you go again," Stephanie says with a chuckle, "messing with these classic sayings."

"It's too many cooks spoil the broth," I correct Janet.

"Maybe your people made broth – chicken soup," she says with a flounce, her bright blue eyes twinkling. "Mine made brew. My grandfather had a booming business during Prohibition. He cooked hootch on a homemade still."

I try to laugh but can't pull it off. I hope they can't tell I'm not in my usual good spirits and don't enjoy the silly banter as I usually do.

Before we leave, Janet pulls me aside. "What's wrong? You're not yourself."

Of course I tell her.

"Take the meds," she urges me. "Why the hell not? Do whatever it takes to feel better. What's your problem? You wouldn't treat a patient like this. Depression requires treatment as much as a bone fracture or a thyroid condition. You wouldn't neglect those conditions. Why the double standard?"

And so, because I adore her as a friend and respect her as a professional – and in my heart, I know she's right – I take Janet's advice.

They say it takes a few weeks for these pills to kick in, but on the way home I fill the prescription, take one, and within hours I feel an effect. A shift. My spirits have lifted. By the next day, I can smile, move my body with ease. Life is back into perspective; it's manageable. My old confidence is back.

Robyn hears it immediately on the phone. "You sound better, Til. It's you again."

"When are you coming back to work?" the nurses had asked me at lunch and for the first time since my surgery, I can see myself returning to the hospital, being a nurse again. Is it friendship, family, meds, or simply "tincture of time" that has healed me?

I even hunt down the Cardiac Patient Handbook that I'd left under a pile of unread newspapers and take another look:

"Some patients find their sex drive is low during the recovery period after cardiac surgery,"

That's rich. How about nonexistent? I thought upon reading that when I came home from the hospital, but now, ten weeks later . . .

I feel differently. I read on: "If you are able to climb two flights of stairs without fatigue or shortness of breath, you may resume sexual intercourse . . . the best positions are on your side or with the person who has had surgery on the bottom . . ." Mmm . . . Sounds doable. I look at Ivan and think it over.

At dinner, we eat leftover chicken soup. Max watches me with interest, an idea in his eyes. "What would happen," he asks, pointing his fork at my chest, "if I were to open up that incision of yours and pop a matzah ball in there?"

For some reason, I find this hysterically funny. We all do. Is it the goofy joke, the medication, or life itself pulling me back in? I don't know, but what fun it is to laugh again!

16

SPINNING WHEEL . . . GOT TO GO 'ROUND

By mid-November my blue funk is completely gone. The spring is back in my step. Energy and joy have returned. I'm a player, back in the game.

First thing, I reach out to friends I've been avoiding or to whom I was rude or unfriendly. Instantly forgiving, they welcome me back and we plan lunches and get-togethers. Next, I reconnect online, ploughing through my backlogged inbox, getting in touch with colleagues, even enjoying silly email jokes sent to me, like "Surprising Animal Sex Facts" with such arcane tidbits as "a snail's genitals are located in its head," "a pig's orgasm lasts thirty minutes" and "the swan is the only bird with a penis." (That's "some pig!" — the phrase woven into the spider's web to describe Wilbur in *Charlotte's Web* — comes to mind.) I have arisen from the couch and turned off the TV, though occasionally I still indulge my guilty pleasure of the glamorous L.A. tattoo artist, Kat Von D., who has taught me how body art can tell a story, commemorate an event, or express a belief. This may be obvious to anyone who has a tattoo, but it's helped me to grasp the meaning of mine. My scar tracks my journey from feeling wounded to being healed. This cracked, broken place has made me stronger. I won't be covering it. I'll wear open necklines – my big reveal. I'm going to rock this scar!

I've rejoined the local gym for physical workouts and the synagogue for spiritual ones. I've passed the major milestones – off all painkillers, made it through my first sneeze, have resumed driving, and now into vigorous exercise.

"Why not start out slow?" Ivan asks when I tell him about my new spinning classes where the teacher pushes us to our limit.

Ivan – always a model of balance and common sense! But gentle aerobics or restorative yoga is not what my body craves. It needs to stride, run, stomp, jump, climb, push, kick, dance, hurl, heave, and roar, because now I can!

He shakes his head wearily. "Does the phrase *everything in moderation* mean anything to you?" Having lived with me so many years, he knows the answer.

When the cardiac rehab centre calls to tell me there's an opening in the upcoming class, I turn it down, but only because I have devised my own rehab program.

At the gym I have found the teacher and class for me. It's cycling on a stationary bicycle to pumped-up, high-voltage music – everything from rock, pop, classical, country, techno, to disco. Zooming from head-banging Metallica to bubblegum "Build Me Up, Buttercup" to Amy Winehouse's "Rehab," Steve switches to "You Lift Me Up . . ." and Josh Groban's soaring tenor voice pours over our sweaty, panting bodies.

"Nice work, Karima," he calls out. "Faster, Tilda! Way to go, Dejeanne! You can do better, Massimo, push yourself!" Without warning, he changes it up to group karaoke with Carly Simon's "You're So Vain." When he makes his way over to me and points the microphone in my direction, I find myself belting out, "You prob- ably think this song is about you" for the whole class to hear.

"Let me ask you to do one thing," says Steve, who offers personal reflections along with fitness tips. "When you're pushing yourself and you're in pain, go toward it. Push through it. Another thing — say out loud and clear what you're feeling: 'It hurts!' It will help you to express what you feel, identify your emotion."

"How'ya doing?" he asks us a few minutes later with a big grin that's a heads-up that something bad is coming. "Feeling good? In the groove?" We nod, riding hard, in the zone, unable to answer. "If you're in your comfort zone . . . Get out of it!"

He's as good as any of those TV New Age motivational speakers — and, with his middle-aged but firm butt and glistening baldness, to me anyway, much hotter. Afterward, I compliment him on the class and tell him about my heart surgery.

He looks surprised. "Aren't you a bit young for that?"

That's the perception of cardiac surgery, but not the reality. "It can happen to anyone, at any age. Everyone should see their family doctor for checkups."

And I've made a surprising discovery: exercise is an ideal time to pray. Yes, at last, I do permit myself to say and to feel prayers of gratitude.

I pick up Max after school and we drive to our favourite Middle Eastern spot for takeout shawarma and falafels in pita, all dripping with hummus, tahini, and hot sauce. (The diet component of my cardiac rehab program will start soon.) It's great to be driving again, behind the wheel, master of my destiny!

"Don't forget your seat belt, Mom," he says, buckling me in. "We wouldn't want anything to happen to Dr. David's hard work now, would we?"

As I'm about to leave my parking spot, I see that I'm boxed in. The guy blocking me gets out of his car and patronizingly tries to guide me out of the tight spot he put me in. The nerve of him! "I wouldn't have this problem if you'd left me enough space," I shout at him and he gives me the finger in return. I honk back at him. "I just had open-heart surgery, you know!" I call out as I turn the wheel left then right, then left, inching out slowly.

Max is enjoying this scene. "Still playing the cardiac patient card, I see." He looks proud of me. "News flash: Mom's back!"

"I can't stay long," Stephanie warns us as she arrives at the bagel shop early on Sunday morning. She takes up her bar stool seat at our high, round "reserved" table. She rests her knapsack on a nearby table and stashes a lumpy, large plastic bag underneath. "I'm beat. I'm going to have to eat, knit, and run."

"Shorty's in a hurry again," Janet chortles. "Not *Eat, Pray, Love,* it'll be Work, Bagel, Sleep."

"Is it legit for me to attend this meeting when I haven't worked?" I ask, suddenly feeling shy, all rested from sleeping in my bed and they've been working all night at the hospital. I feel like I haven't earned my place at the bagel shop this morning.

"We'll overlook it this time," Stephanie warns, "but if you want to keep your spot, you better come back to work soon."

We weave back and forth from our usual topics of mortgages, motherhood, and menopause, wayward teenagers, and bladder control issues (a more common problem in our demographic than you might think), and of course, we soon come full circle, back to the ICU. After finishing their bagels, they pull out their knitting.

I recall how each knit and purl threatened to number my days and myself, a dropped stitch. Fear made my mind so out of control that I imagined them like *tricoteuses*, the knitters who frequented the public beheadings of aristocrats in Paris during the French Revolution. Most notorious of all was Madame DuFarge in the Dickens's classic *A Tale of Two Cities* (another classic that, coincidentally, Janet is currently reading). She knitted and laughed as heads dropped from the guillotines. It had felt like mine was on the chopping block, too. (This must be where the phrase *spinning yarns* comes from, and I admit I do have a runaway imagination. Luckily, I have sensible friends to bring me back to earth.)

I help Jasna untangle a ball of yarn.

"Hey, Tillie, you were MIA there for a while," Janet says. "We were going to put out an Amber Alert on you. Oh, I bet you were in the *sin-ee-gogue* for the Jewish Holidays, right?"

Under my tutelage, they have learned about the Jewish holidays in sound bytes — and edible bites, too: Fried potato pancakes at Chanukah represent oil in a lamp found in a synagogue desecrated by an enemy army. In late winter, there's the Festival of Purim when here, in this bagel shop, they've sampled the three-cornered prune or poppy-seed cookies Eric bakes to symbolize the pointed hat of a would-be assassin whose plot to annihilate the Jewish people was foiled by Queen Esther. They know the reason that the bagel shop is closed at Passover is because only unleavened bread is allowed in remembrance of the haste with which the Israelites fled Egypt to escape the Pharaoh who tried to kill their first-born. What a joyous history my people have. *Bon appetit!*

"Hey, what foods do you eat for Rosh Hashanah?" Janet asks.

"Apples dipped in honey to symbolize a sweet year ahead."

"What about Yom Kippur? What's on the menu for that one?"

"Nothing! We fast all day to atone for our sins."

"Well, you better get cracking. You've got a lot of work to do."

"Yup, and a lot to be grateful for," I say, looking around this very table.

Stephanie reads my mind, or at least my emotions.

"Don't get all sentimental on us now. We're here for bagels, not bawling," she says, trying to be stern with me. "So, are you feeling better these days?" She peers closely at me, but they all see that I am. You're back to yourself. Your spark has returned, they all say. There's light in your eyes again. "You're looking good, Til," she says.

We move quickly from the bagels and banter, from the gossip and girl talk, to our never-ending inquiry into our work, what it means, how we can do it better. We never tire of talking about where nursing takes us, what we see there, and what we are privileged to be able to do for people in need.

In her quiet, understated manner, Jasna tells us about her night on the Rapid Respond Team.

"I was called to consult on the floor. It was a woman, two days post-op. I assessed her and she was dry, so I gave her fluids and did blood work — little things — maybe it was just the close attention — but she really perked up. I love when patients get better," Jasna says with a sigh that makes it obvious she's thinking of the others. "Then I went to see another patient I was concerned about and ended up spending most of the rest of the night with him. When I got there, he was lying in bed, vomiting coffee grounds, blood-streaked bile. He was confused, mumbling to his wife in Serbian, but I could understand him because it's my background, too."

"What did you do?" I asked.

"I sat him up, cleaned him, got an order for an X-ray, drew some blood work — blood cultures, too, because he had a very high temp, started a bigger IV, gave him fluid and he perked right up. I spoke to him in Croatian and he responded appropriately."

"But how did he understand you?" I ask.

"It's the same language, silly," she says, grinning at me for not knowing that and without meaning to, unintentionally reminding me how little we know about cultures other than our own. "Anyway, technically, I could have signed off on him because his condition had improved, but I was still worried because he was slightly rest-less and his vitals weren't rock solid – subtle things that could easily get missed on the floor. I spoke with the doctor about whether we should bring him to the ICU. We decided to monitor him closely on the floor today and I'll follow up on him when I'm back tonight." She looks satisfied with her night's work and returns to the scarf she's knitting.

Jasna is as accomplished a knitter as the others but hasn't mastered the knack of knitting and talking at the same time like the other two. Stephanie is busy with her usual pair of colourful socks, and Janet has another baby blanket on the go, this one in soft, pistachio-coloured yarn.

"How do you know so many babies?" I used to tease her as I watched her produce blanket after blanket. That was before I found out that she donates them to orphanages or gives them to single mothers on welfare who in all likelihood don't knit for their babies.

"I like to know the gender before I get started on the blanket," she says. "Ultrasounds are so detailed, believe me, they know, but the patient I had last night, his daughter who is pregnant and com-pletely on her own – the Baby Daddy left her – three weeks away from delivery – wouldn't tell me. Her mother died a few years ago and her father is having a bone marrow transplant. It's been a rough go for all of them, so this one is for the new baby."

"It's a beautiful blanket," I say, fingering the lacy pattern. "Doesn't it bother you that the baby is going to pee on it, spit up on it?"

"Life is for living. We should use our treasures, not save them."
Her fingers fly over the silky wool, making the blanket blossom like
a living thing, filling her lap under the table, growing minute by
minute as we sit here talking.

I ask them more about the Rapid Response Team because it fas-
cinates me so much and because knowing expert nurses were
there, waiting in the wings if something had gone wrong with me,
was one of the things that reassured me the most. They all say they
are enjoying this new path their career has taken and find it exciting and satisfying. They plan to stay with it, but only as an adjunct
to their regular shifts in the ICU. They are proud to be adding to the
growing bank of worldwide data that proves that rapid response
teams are saving lives and reducing ICU admissions. But the role
does involve huge additional responsibilities for nurses, and offers
only marginally more pay and little recognition.

"Nursing is not an easy sport," Janet says. "It's for the young.
Maybe *we bees* in the wrong business. One day I'm going to open a
yarn and fabric store for knitters and quilters. I'll serve tea and of
course bagels, too."

"I'm staying," Stephanie says. "*I's* happy being a worker bee. I
like where I am." She's entertained the idea of moving from bedside nursing into teaching or a job with more normal hours but
so far hasn't strayed from the ICU. The Rapid Response Team keeps
her busy along with a new mission she's taken on of spearheading
initiatives to make our ICU more "green," reminding everyone to
turn off lights and finding ways to reduce waste and recycle supplies. Stephanie is not one to sit much, except when knitting.

"*I's* staying put, too," Janet concedes. "The youngsters need us
old farts. That's what I love – passing the torch to the young ones.
They need us. They're still hassled by doctors who don't listen to
them. Sometimes the young'uns themselves don't have the

confidence or the knowledge to speak up in the first place. The
other night a nurse on the floor paged me about a patient whose
blood pressure was low. I asked her what she was planning to do
about it. 'I don't know,' she says, 'but I'm writing it down in the
patient's chart.' What good is that? So, I went for a look-see and
assessed the situation myself. He was an eighty-five-year-old man
with multiple medical problems, who'd been in and out – mostly in
– of the hospital for over a year. He had made his choices, even
gone to the trouble of documenting them, and was adamant that he
didn't want life support or to be in the ICU, but his kids didn't agree.
They wouldn't let him go in peace. When I got to him, he was in the
throngs of dying and –"

"The 'throes,'" I interrupt her.

"What?"

"It's the throes of dying. Go on."

"Well anyways, his sons insisted that everything be done – a full
code – and the wife was persuaded by them to go along, so we
resuscitated him. We brought him down to the ICU, intubated him,
and he's hanging in there, alive – for now, anyway."

"It's reassuring to hear that nothing has changed in my absence,"
I comment dryly but don't allow myself to go to that contentious
subject that usually preoccupies me so much. Instead, I return to the
more upbeat topic of the young, upcoming generation of nurses.
I asked about Shauna, one of the newer ones I'm particularly fond
of. They tell me she's become an amazing nurse. She impressed
me, too, on one of the last shifts I worked. A doctor wrote a hemo-
dialysis order that she didn't agree with. Her patient's blood pressure was low and unstable, so she thought that a different modality,
called SLED,* which removes waste products at a slower, more grad-
ual rate, would be preferable for this particular patient.

---

* SLED stands for slow, low-efficiency dialysis.

"So, I went down to the floor to talk to the resident," Shauna told me. "At first he wouldn't even listen to me, but then he realized that I knew what I was talking about and that he needed to know what I was telling him so that he could tell me what I needed to do," she said in obvious frustration at this conundrum. "In the end, I spelled out the order for him and made arrangements for the change of plan. All he had to do was sign off on it."

I see the good ol' doctor-nurse game plays on . . .

Nurses often know more than they let on or are allowed to put to use. In fact, many are so well educated that their scope of practice could be safely expanded, only to the benefit of patient care. Why can't nurses order a blood test or an X-ray if they have reason to believe they're indicated, or choose a laxative or pain medication for their patient? After all, what's important is not who writes the order but that the right things get ordered and properly done.

"How about you, Jazzy? Any plans to leave?" Janet asks.

"I'm not going anywhere," she says simply. Jasna, a caregiver around the clock, is like many nurses I know: rarely off-duty.

"How is Simone doing? Is she still in the ICU, hanging in there?" I ask them about the young nurse I worked with on my last shift in the ICU.

"Yup, she's doing great," Janet says. "We all assumed she was going to be one of these gung-ho types, you know, the ones who've been a nurse for all of two and a half minutes and are already planning to go back to school to do their master's degree. It makes you wonder who's going to stick around to take care of patients. But Simone says she likes the ICU and that she still has a lot to learn."

She's got that right. We all do.

"Simone was overwhelmed," Jasna says. "All she needed was a little guidance."

"We've taken her under our wing," Janet assures me, looking

even more mother-hen-ish than ever. I can picture her protective
wings spread out over her baby nurse birds, watching over them
and nurturing them until they're ready to fly on their own.

I wish I had been more supportive on that last shift when I
worked with Simone, but I am secretly comforted when I hear that
a newbie is nervous. In time, they will overcome their fear, but it's
a good sign, at least at first. It means they realize what they're taking
on. It's like the Hebrew word for "awe," which also means "fear," as
the Rabbi explained at Rosh Hashanah services. This awe/fear
combination is the awareness of the potential of our actions for
good or harm. There's a popular slogan: "Nursing — making a difference." Yes, but bad nursing makes a difference, too. Harming
someone does, too; *killing* someone makes a huge difference. *Only
good nursing makes things better.*

Then there are the calls to arms to "rally the troops" and "recruit"
and "retain" more nurses. Why the military jargon? It smacks of
coercion yet is in widespread use in nursing circles. Who wants to
be recruited (like a soldier?) or retained (what — against our will?)
to a profession as difficult as this? Why not *attract* people, *support*
them in this challenging career, and *keep* them in it by creating
healthy workplaces? Sounds radical.

"Yes, Tilda, Simone is coming along. We're working with her.
Haven't sent her off the show in tears, yet. She's still a contender,"
Stephanie says.

Janet's got an insider scoop and moves closer. "I found out she
was having boyfriend problems and I told her to dump the guy
because in my humble opinion —"

"There she goes again," Stephanie says.

"He's a bum," Janet gets in her two cents, then proceeds to put
me on notice. "So you see, Tilda, you're not the only one who has
problems. Everybody's got their shit to deal with."

"*Dr. Phyllis* has spoken," I shoot back.

I look around the table. It's true. Everyone has something or someone they're worried about. Jasna's son's seizures are getting worse, more frequent. What must it be like for her and her husband to see their child suffer like that, day in, day out? She is like so many nurses: caring is the reality of their public lives and their private ones, too.

Stephanie is doing well, capably raising two splendid teenaged daughters on her own. She's now well recovered from her own health scare that has made her even more grateful for her good fortune and aware of taking care of her health.

"Goin' for the squeeze next week," she says cheerfully.

She's been diligent about her yearly mammograms ever since her mother died of breast cancer. She's in training for a two-day walk – The Weekend to End Women's Cancers – she does every year to honour the memory of her mother and to raise thousands of dollars for cancer treatment and research. Janet joins her, as captain of the medical team, organizing first-aid stations.

"Easy for you to say," says buxom Janet about our skinny-minny friend. "You've got two fried eggs. Imagine me having to cram my shelf into that machine. Well, there's one good thing about being well endowed – I'll never fall on my face!"

"So, Tilda, when do you think you'll come back to work?" Jasna asks.

"Soon," I say evasively, though not meaning to be. I really don't know.

"Are you ready?" Janet asks, looking me over, sizing up my readiness.

"Almost," I say cautiously. I've been away from work for six months now, since before the start of the summer. Fall has come and gone, now it's winter, but suddenly I feel nervous about returning to the ICU. Not as bad as when I started out, years ago, but whenever I've been away from it, like after each of my ten-month maternity leaves, or even after a long vacation, I get this uneasy feeling, worrying about whether I still have that edge, if I am up to its challenges. It's that fear and awe combo.

"When you get there, you'll get your mojo back," Jasna assures me.

A wave of bagel customers just came in and Eric introduces us, the nurses after night shift. They see us and must think, *Knitting nurses. How sweet.*

I watch my friends' graceful, swiftly moving hands and think of all the lives they've saved with those very same hands that are now occupied with this seemingly trivial, decorative hobby. Those onlookers have no idea the mighty battles these hands have waged. I bet they don't even know that it is nurses like these who would save their lives. If they should be unlucky to land in the hospital, they'd be very lucky to fall into these hands. How do we save this species of nursing from extinction? How to grow more nurses like these and ensure there are enough of them to meet the needs of everyone who needs them, which is everyone, one day?

All I know is, what strengthens me the most is being a nurse.

Robyn had told me that as I was being wheeled into the operating room, I gave her a thumbs-up. "It made me so emotional when you did that," she said. "There you were, taking care of me even at that very moment."

"I don't remember, but that was nice of me. It's what friends do."

"But you weren't just being my friend," she continued. "It was more than that. You were taking care of me, as a nurse would, up to the very last minute that you were able."

"Nurses don't like to ask for help," Stephanie says. "It's so hard for us to be on the receiving side. When the roles get flipped, we feel we've failed, let others down. We're supposed to be the strong ones, taking care of others. It's so ingrained in us to feel this way, but we can get sick, too. We need to be able to ask for help."

Out of the blue, I think of a patient I hadn't thought of in years. I was working on a general surgery floor, absentmindedly giving a bed bath to an elderly women, busy thinking about the next patient I had to bathe, all the meds I still had to give out, and the dressings I had to change. I was distracted, my mind not with the patient I was caring for on what turned out to be one of her last days on earth.

She looked up at me. "I was a nurse, too," she said quietly, "once..."

I looked at her gnarled hands, crisscrossed with blue veins, soft and so worn that the tips were perfectly smooth – her fingerprints almost gone – from years of hard work. Yup, I believed her. If I needed proof, there were those hands.

"I took care of many people . . ." Her voice trailed off.

I nodded. She seemed pleased that I knew who she was.

"Now, nurses are taking care of you," I said, though she had fallen asleep.

I'm having a tidal wave surge of love for these three individuals at this table and for many nurses I know. I'm bursting with pride to be a nurse and to be a part of this world. My rhapsodic musings are abruptly interrupted by Stephanie, who pulls out from under the table the big plastic bag she brought with her.

"What've you got in there?" I ask. "A bunch of dirty uniforms?"

"No. As a matter of fact, it's a present. For you."

It's a stunning, jacket-length sweater coat. Loosely knit with deep, wide pockets, an oversized collar, and shiny, dark green buttons, in black wool, shot through with streaks and flecks of metallic pink, gold, and green. How well she knows my taste. It's thoroughly practical and appropriately bohemian – perfect for a suburban mom and *artiste* wannabe like me. What's best is that it is *handmade*.

"But you always said you were a sock girl, could never commit to a sweater!" I say, getting up to give her a hug.

"For you I can. Winter is coming. It's getting chilly. You have to keep warm for your long walks. What with the puppy you were planning on getting?"

This is all you need, what we all need to have and to be – friends like these.

At home, I look in the mirror and see myself. I'm ready to be a nurse again.

"Great work, Tilda!" Steve calls out to me in my new spot in the middle of the pack, no more hiding in the back row as I did at first. "Go, go, go!" he shouts at us. During the cool-down, he offers advice: "Whatever you do, do it the best you can. If you don't know how to do something, learn it."

I feel better, stronger, fitter than ever. Your chronological age isn't always the same as your real age. Maybe age is like weight. How old you are has a set-point, a mind of its own. Forty is mine. I'm almost fifty but feel forty. When I turned forty, I found my voice and finally felt grown-up. Now I feel neither old nor young, but as I get on in years, I feel younger.

At home in the evening, watching TV with Ivan on the couch, I feel blood flowing through my body to places it never reached before – through my veins, to my earlobes, fingertips, the back of my knees. I feel ready for anything and everything.

I take another quick glance at the Cardiac Patient Handbook.

"The energy expended during sexual activity is approximately equal to that required to climb a flight of stairs," it says. *Why, I can race up and down stairs now!* I recall Dr. David's prescription for sex and the health benefits of lovemaking – and the inspiring example of the super-sexed swine. *Thirty minutes? Watch out, Ivan!*

I feel loving again.

After we drink our coffee and watch the late-night news, I take Ivan's hand. We go upstairs and close the door.

The pig is back.

17

THE DIAMOND RULE

"I'm baaa-aaack!" I announce to everyone at the nursing station.

It feels great to be here. I've been away from work for six months. It's now three months since my surgery and I can run, climb stairs, even lift weights — I'm ready to lift patients. It's early — 0600 hours, more than an hour before the official start of my shift at 0715 hours — but I was so nervous/excited all night, I hardly slept. My jitters melt away in a moment when I am welcomed back with greetings, hugs — and, of course, cake.

When I see Dr. Laura Hawryluck, I discover we have something in common: she was recently a patient and is also newly back, recovering from a knee operation.

"Until you've had surgery, you think you know what pain is, but you don't. I learned so much from being a patient. It's made me a better doctor."

How could that be? She was already one of the best.

Most of the nurses know why I was off work, but one pretends she doesn't.

"Did'ja have a bad case of writer's block?" she teases. "Are you back for more stories?"

Now I have my own story. And they still don't believe I love this place, this work. Though most of them wouldn't admit it, they love it, too — if the way they do it is any indication. Isn't it natural to love what we're good at and to be good at what we love?

Ingrid Daley is in charge today — she and I go *waaayyy* back. I see her at the front desk, bent over the staff list, making up the patient assignments.

"I've kept you as extra today, Tilda," she tells me, "to ease you back in gently." She glances up from this complicated match-making to look at me squarely. "What was it like being a patient?" she asks. "The truth. You must have been te-ri-fi-ed," she says, making it a four syllable word. "Any nurse would be."

I nod my head in agreement; there's no time to tell the full story.

"Hey, welcome back, Sister Shalom Shalof!" calls out Claire, arguably the funniest of the wise-cracking nurses, as she gives me a new nickname and joins us at the nursing station. "I feel a book coming on," she says. "What'll you call this one? *Secrets Within the Bedsheets?* How about *Nurse Under the Knife?*"

They all call out "helpful" suggestions.

"*Cardiac Confidential!*"

"*Nursed!*"

"*Nightingale Down!*"

"You *should* write about this," someone says. "People love to read about doctors and nurses getting a taste of their own medicine. Doesn't it infuriate you when people ask if it's made you a better nurse? As if you have to be sick in order to understand what patients go through."

Here's yet another myth that holds a grain of truth — that you have to go through something yourself in order to understand what someone else is going through. Yes, I do have a better appreciation of what it's like being a patient from having gone through it myself, but the capacity for empathy shouldn't be limited by one's personal repertoire of experience. You can expand that ability with your imagination, by asking a lot of questions, and listening closely.

"How did you prepare yourself for open-heart surgery?" they all want to know.

"The 'before' was the hardest part," I say. "I was scared out of my mind. But the 'after,' recovering at home, was rough, too. Much harder than I expected. But the actual surgery and hospital stay weren't that bad at all. They give you good drugs."

"You *would* say that. It's so you, Tilda. Always looking on the bright side."

Yes, I am a "cockeyed-optimist," but I had to overcome a lot of fear and negativity in order that I could be as positive as I am now.

In the staff lounge, before the start of the shift, Janet looks up from the book she's reading to salute me. "Yo, Tillie! Listen to this." She reads the opening lines.

It was the best of times, it was the worst of times, it was the age of wisdom, it was the age of foolishness, it was the epoch of belief, it was the epoch of incredulity, it was the season of Light, it was the season of Darkness, it was the spring of hope, it was the winter of despair, we had everything before us, we had nothing before us, we were all going direct to Heaven, we were all going direct the other way.

"*A Tale of Two Cities,*" she says. "That sums it up pretty well, wouldn't you say?"

I've travelled to those cities, gone far away and made it back safely to my hometown.

The shift starts. As a roving "extra," I have light duties – restocking the intravenous line cabinet, checking that the arrest cart is fully equipped and functioning properly, and helping anyone who has a busy patient. Truth be told, not having a patient assignment also gives me an opportunity to stroll around the ICU, chat with friends, and catch up on the latest news – a computer workshop I have to attend, another lecture on patient-centred care – and, best of all, the dish and dirt: nurses who left the ICU and why; the lowdown on romances and breakups; updates on who's blissfully pregnant and who's still trying; "secret" affairs and racy scandals galore. (Why would I ever stop working here? This stuff is irresistible!) More than a village, it's a kibbutz. Everyone knows one another's business – and I like it like that.

Later on in the morning, down in the lobby, I even catch sight of Dr. Tirone David, distinguished as ever in his long, immaculate white labcoat, standing in line at Tim Hortons along with the rest of us mild-roast Java drinkers.

"What are you doing here?" he asks, not recognizing me out of context.

"I work here," I remind him. "I'm a nurse in Med-Surg ICU."

He forgot me, which is a good thing. Maybe it means I didn't get preferential treatment after all, which is as it should be. He offers to buy me a coffee, but I treat him to one instead, with my super-duper charged-up Tim Hortons coffee card, a gift from the ICU team.

"How do you feel?" he asks.

Great, I tell him and ask about his arm, which has been surgically repaired to his satisfaction and is back to normal. Eyes lowered, I sip my coffee, blushing at the memory of my confused state and inappropriate fantasies during my anesthesia-and-narcotic-induced stupor.

When I get back up to the ICU, Ingrid rushes over to tell me there's a patient on the way. She had hoped to give me a quiet day to allow me get my groove back, but if I'm up to it, she says, she'd like me to take this assignment.

"She's *sick*, Tilda," Ingrid says but assures me that if I don't feel I can handle the challenge, she can switch things up to give me a "quieter" patient.

"The patient's on the floor, in respiratory distress, deteriorating fast. The Rapid Response Team is on their way up, bringing her to us. What'll it be? Decide!"

Does she realize the compliment she's giving me? To assign a sick patient to a nurse is one of the highest compliments of all, second in rank only to choosing that nurse to care for yourself or a loved one.

"Yes," I say, suddenly pumped. Adrenalin is racing through my body. *Can I handle this?* I think for a split second. *Yes, I can!*

The room is ready, the team is ready. I am ready. I plunge in.

The bed is wheeled in. One glance and I see it's serious. A woman in her thirties is struggling to breathe, her breaths fast and laboured. She's on 100 per cent oxygen. She needs to be intubated and I wonder why she isn't already. I try to hold off judgment and questions until I receive the complete report from the floor nurse.

Again, I pause: *Can I do this? Am I ready? No time for that. Get to work.*

I go back in and in a flash, it all comes back to me.

The patient is vomiting into a basin and I leap to her side to support her head so she doesn't aspirate. Her oxygen saturations are down to 85 per cent. The respiratory therapist is on standby to intubate and I get the drugs needed, but we stop; hesitation hangs in the air. We're in a holding pattern, but why? We are not protecting this patient's airway and breathing – the A and the B that will soon affect the C.[*]

Over the hubbub of all the people who have converged into the room to help, I catch the patient's name – Suzanne – and her diagnosis – pulmonary hypertension.

How I hate this disease! It's a rare condition where the arteries of the lungs become narrow and stiff, causing high pressure in the lungs and enlargement of the heart. It can be managed medically for a while, but eventually the only "cure" is a lung transplant. Meanwhile, she's struggling to breathe and for some reason we're stalling.

"Why hasn't she been intubated yet?" I ask the doctor and nurse from the floor.

"She's refusing it," the doctor says.

"She's terrified of the tube," the floor nurse explains.

She tells me that the doctors have explained to Suzanne and her family that with her condition, intubation carries additional risks: she might not be able to get off the ventilator and is likely to develop complications. An artificial lung may offer a "bridge" until donor lungs become available, but until that can be put in place she needs to be on a ventilator that will breathe for her. She cannot hold out much longer.

"Yes, but she still refuses intubation." As an aside, the floor nurse adds, "I don't blame her. I'd be the same way" and gives an involuntary shudder. "Her family's in the waiting room. They want to come in right away."

I go back to Suzanne and introduce myself, but she doesn't care about my name – only having a sip of water, which I can't give her because she is at risk for aspiration into her lungs. I get to work, assisting the doctor to put in central IV lines, a pulmonary artery

---

[*]   Airway, breathing, circulation – the mnemonic mantra of CPR.

catheter to measure pressures in her lungs, and an arterial line to monitor her blood pressure and draw blood, and helping the respiratory therapist set up equipment to have on standby. *How long can she last like this without crashing?* I take blood samples, call for a stat chest X-ray, do a twelve-lead electrocardiogram, and start my head-to-toe assessment. Suddenly, I stop. It sounds crazy, but I swear I can feel the family's anxiety from the waiting room. I go out there to bring them in and try to prepare them as I guide them down the long hall toward the ICU.

As gently as possible, I say, "You will see lots of machines, flashing lights, and noises . . . it's scary, but it will get easier each time you come to visit."

Once in the room, her three sisters swarm her bed. Her husband and elderly parents retreat to the sides, to let them have their turn to be closest to her right now.

"Why can't she have a sip of water?" one sister demands. "You see how thirsty she is!"

Suzanne grabs my arm and mouths, "Water." Seeing her thirst, my own mouth feels dry, too. I lick my lips and swab hers with a moist washcloth. Her husband unpacks her bag – toiletries, a pair of furry slippers, and a photograph that he places face down – on the top of her bedside table. He tells me about their two young daughters at home, being cared for by his mother. Suzanne was diagnosed with pulmonary hypertension a few months ago, he says. She's been at home on oxygen and an IV medication called Flolan but has deteriorated over the past few weeks.

The sisters recede to let the parents move closer. They tuck in the covers over their daughter's restless body and smooth them out, probably as they did when she was a child, before bed. *What can we do to help?* their eyes beseech. Her sisters tell me that Suzanne is a mother of two young girls. She's a lawyer, a marathon runner. Yes, she was a smoker, once, a long time ago but stopped ten years ago. She takes excellent care of herself and was always healthy, until this.

"That's in her favour," the ICU resident says to them encouragingly, loud enough for the patient to hear, too. "Right now, Suzanne needs antibiotics for her pneumonia and support for her breathing with a ventilator. She can't hold out much longer." I can feel him striving to find that balance of reality and optimism. "It's serious," he says. "A transplant is her only hope."

She's worsening by the moment, before our eyes. Her respiratory rate is fifty to sixty breaths per minute. Her blood pressure is skyrocketing and her pulmonary artery pressures are nearing the triple digits – the highest I've ever seen. She will tire soon – arrest and die if we don't do something. She may die anyway, but this is her only chance at life.

She begs for ice chips and winces from time to time.

"Are you in pain?" I ask. She shakes her head, no. There are drugs for physical pain, but for mental anguish – not so much. "Do you have any questions?"

No. No pain, no questions, just fear. Overwhelming fear.

We have to rule out a blood clot, a pulmonary embolus, or fluid around her lungs. It's risky, but we "go travelling" (nurse speak) down to the CT scanner room. But she can't tolerate lying flat long enough to do the CT, so we return to the ICU without the results of the scan. I start a heparin drip, in case there is a blood clot, and titrate the infusion to keep her blood the proper viscosity. Gary, the technician, arrives to do an echocardiogram at the bedside. She is restless. It's getting harder for her to breathe. She's tiring.

"I had an echo myself recently," I say to distract her. Her eyes widen. Out of the corner of my eye, I see the family listening to every word I say, trying to read me. *Will I be good for their loved one? Will I take as good care of her as they would, if they could?*

"I was a patient, too, and I was scared just like you."

Her eyes widen. The family move closer. They urge her to stay focused, to keep fighting. "You have to try, Suzanne! Be strong!" They are protective of her and wary of me. They want what every family wants: the nurse to work as hard as they would to save their loved one. They're checking me out to see if I know what I'm doing. Am I the nurse who will make things better? "Please, Suzanne, let them put the tube in," they implore her. They grab on to her knees, clasp her hands, smooth her forehead.

She looks at their expectant faces; she can't let them down but doesn't answer.

The ICU team arrives and I join them outside the door to discuss the situation. It makes no sense, someone says. The patient says she wants to live, but she's refusing intubation. She knows she can't have ice chips but keeps asking for them. If she's not mentally competent to make decisions for herself, we are going to have to let the family decide.

Have you never wanted to lose weight but gone off your diet? I want to ask that young resident. Have you never struggled with temptation or fought the seduction of despair? Have you never experienced confusion, ambivalence, or inner conflict?

It may sound strange, but contradictions often make more sense to me than logic.

"She's thinking it over," I say, "trying to come to her own decision."

Back in the room, I increase the rate of the Flolan drip. I check lab results and accordingly adjust the heparin infusion. I swab Suzanne's cracked lips, measure her urine output (low, this hour), keep an eye on her blood pressure, heart rate, and rhythm, and note that her "sats" have dropped into the low eighties. She tries to sleep, but breathing is too demanding for her to be able to rest.

I can't give her sedation to help her sleep because it will slow down her respiratory rate.

Ignoring the messy room, meds drawn up but not yet given, incomplete computer work, charting undone, supplies that need restocking, I pull up a chair and sit down beside her. With only my body and my eyes, without a word, I send her the message, *How can I help you?* I keep quiet. *The less said, the better.*

"What should I do?" she asks, her eyes searching mine for the answer.

"What are you afraid of?" I ask.

"I don't . . . know." She gives a helpless shrug. "I'm . . . scared to death of the tube. That's the . . . worst, isn't it? What if I can't get off it?"

I nod. *I worried about that, too.* "Being on a ventilator can be scary."

"I can't deal with that. I'm . . . so scared . . . Ice . . . please . . ."

"I understand." *More than you know.* I slip a few chips onto her tongue, at this point her desire for them outweighing the risk of aspiration.

She closes her eyes, savouring the slivers of cold. I vicariously enjoy her enjoyment. I've never learned to make a complete separation with my patients, probably never will at this point in my career. I open my heart to her suffering and stay sitting with her, trying to feel, for a few moments, what she's feeling. Perhaps briefly it lessens her burden to share it with another person? Then I decide to do what no textbook, professor, or policy manual would advise. Most will tell you straight out – don't do this.

"I was a patient myself," I start off and then tell her how scared I was and all that I went through. And that I really do understand what she is going through.

Am I crossing a line by speaking so personally? Probably. It's not harmful, illegal, or unethical, but it's *unprofessional. To hell with that. This is war!*

"Before my surgery, I felt just like you do, but I decided to let go and trust the people taking care of me. They kept me comfortable and safe and I promise you the same, whatever choice you make." *I am here to serve you.* Face to face, we speak, heart to heart, just two women – wives, mothers, daughters, doing what it takes to survive. Both on the same side.

Speaking has become too much of an effort, so she motions to write a note. I prop up a clipboard, hand her a pencil, and await the discovery of her thoughts. Words on paper bear a different significance than spoken into the air or produced as digital markings on a computer screen.

feel Like a monster?

The tube is horrible

awake? No!

I could comfort, explain, soothe, or elaborate but stop myself. I could pull away and get busy; it's tempting to do so. I need to organize my medications, get my charting done. Get up, walk away. Instead, I sit still why she ponders these fateful decisions.

"Patient-centred care" is not as easy as it looks.

Keep a distance, they told us in school – we tell one another – but no one can explain how to do that exactly. *Don't get too personal.* Offer *empathy,* not *sympathy,* they advised, but who among us has mastered the ability to calibrate our emotions with a tweak of vocabulary? In order to understand another person you have to open your heart as wide as on an operating table. We have to be so attuned to patients that we are able to offer what *they* need, not

what we want to give. Most ordinary people aspire to The Golden
Rule to treat others as we wish to be treated, but more is expected
of caregivers who must treat others as *they* wish to be treated.
Perhaps it's The Diamond Rule – just as durable and shiny but
not so reflective that you only see yourself in its sheen. Suzanne
scrawls me a note:

Don't know if life is worth this pain
What do you Think?

After she writes each note, she motions for me to get rid of it so
her family won't see. After tossing the last one in the garbage pail,
I go over to the bedside table and on instinct pick up the photograph her husband brought – it's a picture of her daughters – and
bring it over to show it to her. *Here's what we're talking about. These
are the stakes. Have you had enough and want to start saying goodbye
or do you want to keep on fighting?* I reserve all judgment; I am here
to help you achieve your wishes.

For her, this is an existential battle; for us, her answer will be the
blueprint of our care.

Perhaps out of sheer exhaustion, the family's pleading, the
reminder of that photograph, or the force of her innate will to survive, Suzanne nods and whispers, "Yes." We intubate her and at
last, well sedated, she looks comfortable. There is surrender, and
with it peace, in her now-relaxed body. Her family goes home to
rest. Soon, a team will arrive to put the artificial lung in place. It
will buy her time and, if the stars are aligned in her favour, an
unknown family's magnanimity at a time of tragedy will bring new
lungs to give her a chance at life.

"In the meanwhile, you are in good hands here," I whisper to
her.

Your destination is unknown, but we can guarantee you a safe journey.

Toward the end of my shift, I run down to the Cardiovascular ICU to find my nurses, the ones who took care of me. Joy is on and I ask her the question that continues to bedevil me.

"How do you do it?"

Joy thinks for a few moments, keeping her eyes on her patient in the bed a few steps away. When she finally speaks, it is as if she's receiving cues emanating from that person. "I never allow myself to forget that a person's life is in my hands," she says slowly, visibly thinking this through as she speaks. "The surgeon has repaired the heart, and now it's up to me to take it from here. I could never forgive myself if I harmed someone in any way. I always take it seriously and try to do the right thing. I never allow myself to forget that this is someone's loved one. If I imagine how it is for the patient, I know how to care for that person"

There's Maria coming on now, arriving for night shift. She greets me warmly.

"May I give you a hug?" she asks me in her respectful, slightly formal way.

Of course. She puts her arms around me. It was into these very arms that I was delivered when I was in life-threatening danger; she brought me back from the brink. "She watched you like a hawk," Robyn had said. Yes, Maria was the eagle at my back. One of them.

What makes a great nurse? It takes more than knowledge or skill and it's not enough to be *caring* in the sentimental sense of the word. I think of Maria and other nurses like her. Do they love nursing? They probably wouldn't express it like that. Some would laugh off that word; it might make them uncomfortable – but to be a great nurse takes intelligence, energy, imagination, integrity, and at the risk of sounding unscientific and *unprofessional,* I've come to the conclusion that an additional element is required: love. How could you do this work otherwise?

Love is a lot to ask, but there's no way around it.

You have to add love to the mix.

Stir. Shake. Serve.

Epilogue

IN A HEARTBEAT

It's been two years now.

We got a puppy. On purpose I didn't choose a lapdog or a purse pooch. Toby is a big, high-energy border collie and shepherd mix who needs lots of exercise. Intuitively, I knew that by fulfilling his needs, I would be fulfilling mine. He and I walk miles of city streets, explore its green spaces, and hike rugged country trails. We run together, he alongside me, stopping now and again to look up and check on me. *You can do it,* he seems to say, egging me onward, stronger, faster, longer. And when I occasionally need a reminder to be grateful and enjoy each moment, he shows me how and reminds me of my life's purpose.

For years I lived my life, knowing it could be over in a heartbeat. My heart is fixed and healthy now, but I still live with that sense of urgency. This journey has brought me renewed health, a greater appreciation for each day, and the discovery that the set-points for age and weight may be constant, but it's possible to raise your *happiness* set-point. I know I did.

And yes, in retrospect, I guess I did have one of those sought-after "near-death" experiences. I went as close to the edge as you can go and made it back to tell the tale. I didn't find out whether there's life after death, only that there is life *before* death, and I want to live it to the fullest. Yes, I still lose my temper at times, sink into mindlessness, don't meditate or exercise enough, and have a few pounds to lose, but when I get stressed out, my friends, family — and especially my children — keep me in check. Like the other day, I yelled at Max about his messy room — unmade bed, clothes on the floor, wads of used hockey tape, rotting apple cores, etcetera, etcetera. "This place is a pigsty!"

"Well, *you* would know," I thought I heard him mutter under his breath.

"What did you say?"

"Chill, Mom. It's not open-heart surgery."

The kid's got a point.

And when I turned fifty and was feeling both joyful and a touch morose, Harry turned to me and said in his level-headed way, "You've lived half your life, Mom."

If I make it to one hundred in good health, what a gift that will be, but I am willing to forego fewer days in exchange for a natural, dignified end when my time comes.

Ivan wanted to throw me a big birthday bash (not surprisingly, Ivan doesn't do surprises), but what shindig could top open-heart surgery? I already got the best gift.

And yes, I still worry a lot about the health care system, but I believe the vision of quality health care for all is possible. The problems are fixable with the resources we have. It is our expectations that have to be brought in line.

I am lucky. I have no complaints about the health care I received, only praise. Many would claim that I feel that way because I received special treatment: I was an insider, was treated in a world-class hospital, had a brilliant surgeon, expert nurses, a posse of protectors, and a close circle of supportive friends and family. Nothing whatsoever can be concluded about the health care system based on my singular experience and I'm the first to admit I was fortunate — even privileged — but isn't what I received what everyone deserves? It shouldn't require fortune, luck, money, or connections to get what I got — not when it comes to health care. Why can't everyone have great health care?

This is what I still don't understand: why can't we make sure that every human being gets what they need, whether it's open-heart surgery, cancer treatment, mental health care, HIV retroviral agents, pain relief, attention to an ear infection, and, of course, clean water, healthy food, and safety?